Praise for
Farm Sanctuary

"I have always admired the tremendous work of Farm Sanctuary. Farm animals need our ethical consideration, and Farm Sanctuary has played a central role in getting the issue of their plight on the national agenda."
—Wayne Pacelle, CEO of the Humane Society of the United States

"Since Farm Sanctuary first opened its barn doors more than twenty years ago, thousands of animals have been rescued, millions of people have been educated, and countless perspectives have been shifted. Farm animals couldn't ask for a better advocate than Gene Baur."
—Rory Freedman, coauthor of *Skinny Bitch*

"In *Farm Sanctuary* Gene Baur highlights the appalling conditions billions of animals are forced to endure in factory farms—in order to produce more meat more cheaply in the shortest possible time. His descriptions of the courageous battles fought by many individuals to end such practices are touching. Filled with hope, this book is written for all who strive for a more compassionate world—I highly recommend it."
—Dr. Jane Goodall, DBE, founder of the Jane Goodall Institute and
UN Messenger of Peace

"Starting in the 1980s, Gene rescued neglected, abused, and injured animals from the appalling, disgusting conditions at auctions and stockyards. Meet in this insightful book the fascinating animals he saved."
—Dr. Temple Grandin, author of *Animals in Translation*

"In this impassioned book, Baur paints an appealing picture of these shelters and the animals that live there far from the brutality of industrial farming [and] makes a strong case that meat eaters have an ethical responsibility to ensure that the animals the eat have not been abused."
—*Publishers Weekly*

"A stunning indictment of factory farming and the way most Americans obtain their food. . . A life-altering read."

—*Booklist* (starred review)

"Farm Sanctuary is a wonderful and inspiring book—about animals in need of compassion and laws in need of reform. Some of the stories Gene Baur tells will break your heart, and other stories will speak to your deepest convictions. It's a book about appalling cruelty and heroic kindness, and it points the way to a better world."

—Alicia Silverstone

"I have had the opportunity to visit the Farm Sanctuary several times and have never been quite as moved. This book is not only a reflection of what Gene and Farm Sanctuary represent but also an eye-opener to anyone who has been in the dark about the abuse in factory farming and what can be done to prevent it."

—Kevin Nealon

"The factory-farming industries do their best to keep people from knowing the truth about how meat, eggs, and dairy are produced. Gene and Farm Sanctuary deserve high praise for working so hard to educate the public and make the world a more compassionate and humane place."

—Moby

"Gene Baur and Farm Sanctuary have helped to bring the U.S. animal welfare movement into the twenty-first century, winning victories for farm animals that have the support of most Americans—once they learn the truth about industrial animal farming today."

—Peter Singer, author of *Animal Liberation*

"With grace and with guts, Gene Baur tells us how he and a few other animal advocates finally stood up for the rights of farmed animals, how they shook awake a sleeping public, and how animal agribusiness fought them all every step of the way. A great read—the best book on the U.S. movement for the rights of animals used for food."

—Jim Mason, author (with Peter Singer) of *The Way We Eat,* and *An Unnatural Order*

"For both humans and other animals, Farm Sanctuary is as close to the Garden of Eden as we have seen in our lifetimes. Now, with the publication of *Farm Sanctuary*, we can read the story of what went into the Garden's creation."

—Tom Regan, author (with Jeffrey Moussaieff Masson) of *Empty Cages: Facing the Challenge of Animal Rights*

"This book is the most authentic account of the real lives of farm animals, by the St. Francis of our time. There is nobody else in America who could tell the truth about farm animals from such a deep perspective, and at the same time make your heart soar."

—Jeffrey Moussaieff Masson, author of *When Elephants Weep* (with Susan McCarthy) and *The Pig Who Sang to the Moon*

"For years, Farm Sanctuary has been a refuge for cruelly treated animals, rescued from the nightmare world of the factory farm. Now *Farm Sanctuary* is also a beautiful and stirring book, as filled with the spirit of mercy as the place that inspired it."

—Matthew Scully, author of *Dominion*

"Not unlike the great liberationist movements of the past—whether those championed by Susan B. Anthony or Mahatma Gandhi—Gene's profoundly successful efforts should rightly be credited with having created the blueprint for what some would call a utopian call to faith, but is, in fact, the true nature of humanity: pragmatic idealism; to be gentle, compassionate, and truly human. This book is his lyrical testimony to the fact it can, and will be done."

—Dr. Michael Tobias, global ecologist, author, filmmaker, president of the Dancing Star Foundation

"Our culture has supported the alarming growth of environmentally toxic, unbelievably cruel, and ultimately unsustainable factory farms for our animal foods. Gene's engaging book traces how we got here, and the hopeful options we have ahead of us for making healthier and more compassionate choices."

—John Mackey, cofounder and CEO of Whole Foods Market

"If you want to pretend that agribusiness treats farm animals just like members of their own families, then this book isn't for you. But if you want to live a compassionate life, and want your choices to be congruent with your love, then read Gene Baur's excellent *Farm Sanctuary*. You'll be a wiser, stronger, and healthier person for it."

—John Robbins, author *Diet for a New America*

"Agribusiness factory farms subvert democracy and are some of the nation's worst polluters. This book shows how they also treat animals with unspeakable cruelty. It is a compelling testament to the need to civilize this industry and end its radical practices for producing meat, dairy, and eggs."

—Robert F. Kennedy Jr.

FARM
Sanctuary

Changing Hearts and Minds
About Animals and Food

GENE BAUR

A TOUCHSTONE BOOK
Published by Simon & Schuster
New York London Toronto Sydney

Touchstone
A Division of Simon & Schuster, Inc.
1230 Avenue of the Americas
New York, NY 10020

First Touchstone trade paperback edition November 2008

TOUCHSTONE and colophon are registered trademarks of Simon & Schuster, Inc.

Photo credits:
© Farm Sanctuary/Derek Goodwin: pp. 36, 53, 79, 125
© Farm Sanctuary/Jo-Anne McArthur: p. 144
© Blanche Johnson-Baransky: p. 165
All other interior photos © Farm Sanctuary

For information about special discounts for bulk purchases, please contact Simon & Schuster Special Sales at 1-800-456-6798 or business@simonandschuster.com.

Designed by Jan Pisciotta

Manufactured in the United States of America

10   9   8   7   6   5   4

ISBN-13: 978-0-7432-9158-3
ISBN-10:   0-7432-9158-1
ISBN-13: 978-0-7432-9159-0 (pbk)
ISBN-10:   0-7432-9159-X (pbk)

To my parents,
Gene and Kay Baur,
for their abiding love and support

There is not enough darkness in all the world to put out the light of even one small candle.

—Robert Alden

Contents

Introduction

Opening the Gate

About eight miles along Route 23, just west of the village of Watkins Glen in the Finger Lakes region of New York State, you crest the brow of a hill and see a glistening lake and green valleys spread before you. A county road sign directs you to turn left onto Aikens Road, which soon becomes a dirt lane bordered by trees that lead to the ten-thousand-acre Sugar Hill State Forest. This forest was cleared to create farmland in the 1800s, but by the Depression of the 1930s farmers could no longer make a living—partly because the valuable topsoil had eroded or washed away—so New York State repurchased the land and replanted it with the trees you see there today.

Following that dirt road around a corner, you leave the forest and the land opens to reveal red barns of various sizes, one white house, and grassy fields. Walking from the parking lot up the rutted path to the entrance, you'll see what you imagine a farm should look like—the kind many of us thought of as we sang "Old McDonald Had a Farm" as children. There are pastures and haybines and balers, manure spreaders and tractors, parked in covered barns or being pulled or driven by farmhands. Much of the year, you can see cows and sheep grazing on the hillsides, while nearer to the barns you can spot pigs rooting in the soil and wallowing in mud holes. The roosters keep a careful eye on the hens as they peck at the soil, groom, cluck, and enjoy the sun. The smell of cut grass and the aroma of wildflowers from the meadows are in the air. There's something unusual about this farm. It differs from most "modern" farms in the United States. For one thing, this farm welcomes visitors. Not far from the main entrance are three bed-and-breakfast cabins where guests can stay and a large building nearby that's called the People Barn.

But the surest indication that this farm is different is a sign by the

gate: YOU ARE NOW ENTERING THE ANIMALS' SANCTUARY. PLEASE REMEM-
BER THAT YOU ARE A GUEST IN THEIR HOME. This is the way into Farm
Sanctuary, which I co-founded in 1986, and which has since grown from
an idea into a national organization and, I hope, into a growing movement of conscience.

A New Kind of Farm

Our idea was to help prevent "factory farming" and give refuge to its
victims, especially the animals so weak or sickly that even the slaughterhouses did not want them. Over the last two decades, Farm Sanctuary
has rescued and cared for thousands of animals. Most were sick, abused,
or left for dead. Others were abandoned by farmers unable to cope with
the demands of their business. Some were rescued after a hurricane or a
tornado, while several escaped from slaughterhouses and needed a place
of safety. Goats, pigs, sheep, cows, chickens, turkeys, geese, ducks, and
the occasional donkey and rabbit have found their way to our sanctuaries in rural New York, about twenty miles from the city of Ithaca, and in
Orland, California, north of Sacramento.

With over a dozen barns at each shelter, hundreds of acres of pasture,
and round-the-clock attention, every sanctuary animal receives the best
of care. For the first time in their lives, animals who have known only the
worst of the world—fear and isolation and pain—suddenly find themselves in clean, spacious, straw-filled barns, getting their first taste of
nourishing food, veterinary care, and human compassion.

Farm Sanctuary is unusual not only because the animals who live
there have been removed from the food chain—they're no longer being
fed and raised for profit or shipped to slaughter once they've reached a
certain weight or age. We're unusual because at the shelter the animals
are free to come and go from the barns and the pastures as they please.
Almost all of what you'll see on a typical day at Farm Sanctuary has
vanished from the American landscape, just like most traditional family
farms. Although it's been a while since most Americans had any real connection with farm life, many of us still have romantic notions of how our
food is made. We think of small family farms where hardworking people

plow the fields, care for animals in barnyards and pastures, and scratch out a difficult but honorable livelihood.

Early on we realized that our role as a refuge could be only a small part of what had to be done. We knew we could rescue or house only a tiny fraction of the billions of animals killed for food in the United States. We knew we had to go "upstream" and stop the cruelty at its source, to reduce the number of abused, injured, or sick animals who came our way. As a result of Farm Sanctuary's efforts over two decades, stockyards and slaughterhouses have been convicted of cruelty to animals, laws have been passed banning abusive factory farming practices, and national news stories have begun to expose the cruelty of industrialized animal agriculture. At the same time, thousands of suffering animals have been rescued from abuse, and given a decent life.

The reality is that over the past fifty years farming has become a mega-industry worth hundreds of billions of dollars each year. Today animals raised for food are confined indoors, away from the fields and the sun, into concentrated animal feeding operations (CAFOs), or more accurately factory farms. What makes them factories is that the animals are kept in vast sheds akin to warehouses. Their lives are highly controlled, and the processes of feeding, watering, treatment, and waste removal are heavily mechanized. Far from being treated as individuals with needs, feelings, and desires, as countless researchers and centuries of firsthand experience have demonstrated, the animals have become merely like so many car parts, units of production. Cows, pigs, sheep, chickens, ducks, and turkeys are confined by the hundreds and thousands in cages, crates, or crowded pens. They are fattened with antibiotic-laced feed and bred to grow big and fast or to pump out milk or their young until they are killed and sent to slaughter, too. The most marketable parts of their bodies—breasts on broiler chickens, rear ends on pigs—are now so outsized that many of the animals have trouble standing, let alone walking. Millions are starved, mutilated, or even discarded. The vast majority don't reach adulthood. This is the reality of the nearly ten billion animals who are raised and slaughtered for food in the United States every year. Their lives are filled with pain, confusion, and loneliness. They go to their deaths having never once experienced anything resembling human kindness.

Abused and bullied at every turn, animals in factory farms are denied the opportunity to express the natural behaviors you see every day at Farm Sanctuary. In this book, I'll describe the roots of factory farming, why I believe it is representative of so much that is wrong with the way we view the natural world and other animals, and why it is an affront to decent and honorable farming. I am well aware that since the dawn of agriculture, roughly ten thousand years ago, people have been raising and slaughtering animals for food, clothing, and other purposes. For nearly all of that time, most of the population was involved in raising animals and tending crops. We understood where our food came from, worked with the land and the animals, and often lived closely connected to cows, pigs, sheep, goats, and chickens (and sometimes in the same quarters with them).

I also want to introduce you to some of the remarkable individual animals who have passed through the gates of Farm Sanctuary's shelters. For some of you, the word *individuals* applied to farm animals may seem strange. We may be comfortable with the idea that the cats and dogs in our homes have personalities or preferences and are part of our family, with their own inherent worth and needs. But we may wonder whether chickens or cows or sheep are the same. We tend to think of them in generalities—herds and flocks—and find it hard to imagine that one chicken may be docile while another is sociable, or one turkey is shy and another showy. In part through the influence of the factory farming mind-set, we no longer *see* the animals as the individual beings they are—let alone allow them to live the lives nature meant for them.

Some of those who have suffered the most from the industrialization of farming over the last two generations have been the farmers themselves. For so many of them, farm work has become factory work. They have been forced into following an economic paradigm that has increased the already considerable pressures of agriculture, sometimes to the breaking point. I have been saddened by the desperation of family farmers as they struggle to do the right thing by the animals they raise in the face of a system that treats both humans and animals as expendable commodities. I know that many of them do not like what has happened to their profession and culture, and I understand the constraints under which they operate. This book will give you a window into the problems they are up against and offer some ideas of how farming and our food system could be different.

Some of what you read in this book will be disturbing, perhaps even depressing. Once you learn about what happens in factory farms, the knowledge can seem so horrific or overwhelming that you want to turn away or pretend not to know. I can understand that, and often myself have wished I didn't have to think about the horrific violence done to animals. I've witnessed staggering brutality to animals and to people, and I've been threatened on many occasions. But bad situations don't simply resolve themselves when we look away. When we face issues, remarkable things can happen. That's why, in spite of the appalling things that I have seen with my own eyes, I remain optimistic that the situation will change.

In an ideal world, there would be no need for Farm Sanctuary. There would be no factory farms or stockyards, and cattle, pigs, chickens, and other farmed animals would not be abused. They would be free to feel the sun and the breeze, scratch at the earth, and generally enjoy life. Human beings have a great capacity to act with sensitivity and compassion, as well as a frightening ability to disregard the feelings of others. The more we act with indifference and cruelty, the more pervasive and defining these qualities become in our world. But when we behave with understanding and kindness, these qualities can spread and flourish.

This, then, is a book of hope. A book of Hope the pig. And Hilda the sheep, Opie the steer, Marmalade the hen, and all the other extraordinary animals from whom I've learned so much over the years. They all came through our front gates and in their own way transformed us by sharing their resilience, their spirit, and their varied and distinctive personalities. Even though we cannot rescue every farmed animal in need, we feel that every animal at Farm Sanctuary is an ambassador for millions, indeed billions, of others. Being in their company allows us to acknowledge our relationship with them, and with all of the animals with whom we share the earth.

This is their story, as it is ours. Just as Farm Sanctuary opened its gates and our hearts to them, I hope you, too, will open your heart and follow where your conscience leads.

PART ONE

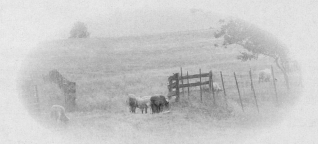

From the
Ground Up

CHAPTER ONE

The Road to Lancaster

You know when it's morning on the farm: the roosters tell you. Usually well before dawn they welcome the new day, as if saying, "We're here." At daybreak, staff workers open all the barn doors, more than a dozen at each shelter. Everybody gets fresh food and water, and health care rounds begin soon after. Any of the animals on a treatment regimen receives his or her shots or pills, has a foot wrap or splints changed, IVs attended to or wounds dressed.

By eight o'clock, the cleaning crews are getting to work. Barn by barn they shovel out old straw into barrels and empty them in the manure spreader, which will be busy later in the fields. Then, as the sun gets higher overhead, the day-to-day work of the farm begins: fixing tractors if they've broken down, reattaching barn doors that have come off their hinges, ordering feed or fencing, and, in season, cutting hay. Pasture by pasture, the animals are monitored to make sure they're all doing well. Those with special needs—fears, diseases, or discomfort from aging, wounds, or illnesses from which they're recovering—get checked individually. If a pasture has been eaten down, a gate is opened and the sheep or cows or goats move into a new one. Their excitement is palpable.

Midmorning to afternoon, school groups, families, and individuals arrive to visit with the animals. As the day progresses, calls come in about cases of farm animal cruelty or requests to take in rescued animals. While the shelter staff manage the farm, the office staff work on legislative initiatives, answer questions from our members and other concerned citizens, research and produce educational and campaign materials, and manage advocacy campaigns around the country.

Around dusk, the animals come back to their barns and settle into the new straw. Once it's clear that everyone is inside, the main doors are closed. Smaller doors that give the larger animals access to the outside aren't closed unless it's a frigid week in Watkins Glen. On warm nights, the bigger barn doors remain open so the cattle, sheep, and pigs can come and go as they please. Since the birds need to be protected from predators when evening comes, their barns are closed. In the summer, sundown can be very late in the day, around nine o'clock. On nights such as these, the cows and the pigs may lounge at the base of trees as the heat of the day subsides. Often, they'll sleep under the stars until the roosters let them know that dawn is about to return.

The Family Business

I wasn't raised on a farm. In fact, I spent my childhood almost as far from the culture of farming as you can get in the United States. I was born in Los Angeles and grew up in the Hollywood hills, in the shadow of the famous Hollywood sign, the oldest of six kids. Like many children, I was drawn to animals. In the hills surrounding Griffith Park (four thousand acres of oak trees and wild sage that's the largest municipal park in the country), which was near our family's house, I saw many wild animals, including deer, coyotes, skunks, raccoons, gophers, and snakes. I remember finding a coyote den on a hillside covered with brush, seeing the antlers shed by deer in our backyard, and visiting frogs in a nearby pond in Canyon Park. In the way of children, I was curious about these other creatures and wanted to know more about them. I would collect the frogs and bring them home and place them carefully in a small pond I had dug in the backyard. Unfortunately, the frogs all died, and I learned my first lesson about wild animals—that it's usually best to let them be.

My mother, like her mother, always had a tender spot for animals. Over the years, my family cared for several companion animals as well as various dogs who wandered around the neighborhood. The first to capture my heart was Tiger, a kitten I adopted when I was about ten, who became one of my best friends. I wanted him to come into the house, while my parents, without much success, wanted him to stay outside. I loved hugging Tiger and was awed by his ability to leap and climb. I was especially happy when he jumped to the top of the bunk bed to sleep with me. Then Tiger got sick. I remember my mother talking on the phone to the veterinarian about me: "He's got an emotional attachment to this cat, so we've got to try to save it." Even though the vet did his best, it was Tiger's time. When he died, I was devastated.

I think everyone has the capacity to experience compassion and empathy for animals, but most of us have it "adulterated," as my friend Jim Mason, an attorney and animal rights pioneer who was raised on a farm in Missouri, calls growing older. But some people remain particularly sensitive to animals, and I am one of them. Even then, I felt Tiger's loss particularly keenly.

It wasn't only the animals who enchanted me, it was also where they lived. As a child, I loved running through the hills in the shade of the tall trees. I wasn't very old, however, when houses around us expanded, as did their driveways, and the stately trees that used to stand in our neighborhood were cut down. The neighbors built walls, and then built them higher, which kept any "undesirables" out. But it also disrupted the natural habitats of the animals who called those hills home. One of my first memories is of an injured deer caught in a fence in a neighbor's backyard.

What happened in my parents' neighborhood near Griffith Park happened all over the country. Not only did we decide to take up more space, but there were many tens of millions more of us to do it. Suburban homes and subdivisions overtook farmland and wilderness areas, confining both humans and animals in artificial ecosystems, where one could be isolated from the other.

Even though I loved my cat and enjoyed the wild animals I encountered, I did not give a thought to the animals on my plate, and my family ate a standard American meat-centered diet. This was the case until a conversation I had as a teenager with my mother's mother. I often visited my grandmother's house in the Eagle Rock section of Los Angeles, about ten minutes away from my family's home, to help her around the house and with her garden. My grandmother shared my interest in animals and used to feed and take care of strays in her neighborhood. One day, she told me about how veal calves were taken from their mothers soon after birth and chained in crates for their whole lives, unable even to turn around. I was stunned. I thought of the wild animals near my home. Even though they were themselves being hemmed in by human development, at least they had some degree of freedom. I hated to be boxed in, and I felt for those who did not have that freedom, too. It seemed wrong and an affront to common decency to take away the calves' ability even to walk, let alone run.

After I learned how veal was produced, I returned one day from school and found my mother had made chicken for dinner. Suddenly, instead of "meat," I saw the body of a headless bird on a plate, on his or her back. Instead of a tasty meal, I saw an animal with wings and legs who had been killed, plucked, and broiled for me. For a time I stopped eating meat, but later I returned to the omnivorous diet of the rest of my family and friends. I also had a connection to animals through my father's family. My last name means "farmer" or "peasant" in German, and my father's mother grew up on a farm in Germany. My father talked about how she would milk the cows every morning, and it clearly lay deep within her consciousness. When she succumbed to Alzheimer's disease in later years, she would suddenly shout that she needed to go out and milk the cows.

My father was the youngest child of German immigrants, and the only one born in the United States. He grew up in L.A. and attended Loyola Marymount University on a baseball scholarship, where he also enrolled in the air force ROTC program. After my father returned from the air force, he and my mother got married, and my father joined his family's business, which was hotel management. My mother also grew up in L.A. and first met my father when they attended grammar school together. She had a full-time job raising me and my five siblings. My mother impressed upon me that there are two primary human motivators—fear and love—and the lesson has stuck.

Family businesses such as my father's were modeled after family farms. A large number of children provided on-site labor for the enterprise as they got older, and that was what happened in our family. As a teenager, I would help my father in the hotel by cleaning or moving furniture. I often think that hotel work prepared me for running a sanctuary—and not only because I moved from cleaning toilets to shoveling manure out of barns and from moving beds to preparing bedding! A family working together and the discipline of looking after guests every day could apply as well to an animal sanctuary as to a hotel.

My father was a smoker. For decades after World War II, catchy commercials and the ubiquity of cigarettes in movies and on television helped romanticize and sell them to a public that associated smoking with sophistication, glamour, and relaxation. The tobacco industry was only too happy to use the media to create positive feelings about cigarettes, and employed doctors and even Ronald Reagan, then an actor, to promote them. But even before I became a teenager, I knew that cigarettes weren't good for you, and my first attempt at activism was to gather my siblings together to try to prevent our father from smoking. We hid his cigarettes and urged him to quit. It worked. He was motivated to be there for us, which certainly benefited his health and well-being, as well as ours.

Decades later, as he approached his seventieth birthday, my father had a heart attack and ended up in the hospital. His arteries were clogged with plaque as a result of all the animal fat he had eaten over the course of his life, and they needed to be opened up. I called the hospital to check on how my father was doing and was shocked and upset to learn that he was being fed bacon and eggs for breakfast. I asked to talk to the doctor, but in spite of my repeated requests, he wouldn't get on the phone. I was angry. "Is this the 'come back and see us' diet?" I asked the nurse who spoke to me. How could a heart patient in the hospital be given foods known to increase the risk of heart disease? It seemed ignorant and irresponsible, and the doctor's refusal to provide an explanation was disconcerting.

After his heart attack, my father picked up a book by Dr. Dean Ornish, who directs the Preventive Medicine Research Institute in Sausalito, California. After reading through it, my father followed Dr. Ornish's suggestions. He stopped eating meat and started eating more grains, vegetables, and other plant foods. One year later, he walked and completed the Los Angeles Marathon. (Since then, he's gone back to eating a more standard American diet—but I'm still working on him!) His heart attack was the wake-up call he needed to live a healthier lifestyle . . . and thank goodness that call didn't come too late.

From Family Farm to Big Agriculture

Just as big tobacco spends billions of dollars to sell us its products, big agriculture (the meat, dairy, and egg industries) is spending untold sums to create positive feelings about its products. Consumers are subjected to relentless advertising campaigns featuring actors, musicians, sports stars, and even people in the government eating and promoting various animal food products. However, as with the cigarette industry, health risks and other problems associated with fast-food hamburgers and other unhealthy animal products are becoming apparent. Unease over industrialized animal agriculture is growing, much as concern over the impacts of tobacco on our health emerged in recent decades. And factory farming is a huge part of the problem.

Industrial farming is now the dominant model of raising animals for food in the United States, Europe, and other developed countries—and, increasingly, in poorer regions as well. How did the United States—whose agrarian identity Thomas Jefferson and other Founding Fathers championed and whose "embattled farmers," as Ralph Waldo Emerson wrote in "Concord Hymn," "stood / And fired the shot heard round the world"—become the hegemonic agribusiness juggernaut it is today?

It was the beef industry that pioneered industrial farming, specifically the five large meatpacking companies—Armour, Swift, Morris, Wilson, and Cudahy—in the latter half of the nineteenth century. Around the same time, the completion of the railroad network from the Atlantic to the Midwest and beyond allowed cattle (an industry term that includes males, both bulls and steers, as well as females) to be transported to, and beef delivered from, Chicago's Union Stock Yards to cities throughout the country for the first time. The Union Stock Yards, which opened at the end of the Civil War in 1865, towered over all previous livestock operations. By 1900, four hundred million animals had been slaughtered and processed in a vast complex containing not only meatpacking facilities and slaughterhouses but also hotels and restaurants, and which covered a full square mile in downtown Chicago. Inside the slaughterhouses, workers turned live animals into meat using the conveyor-belt, factory-line model that inspired Henry Ford when he began making cars in mass quantities.

This is one point where farm work became factory work. Each employee was responsible for only one facet of the processing—for example, slicing a particular body part for a specific cut of meat. He would repeat this motion over and over, thousands of times a day. In this way, a highly skilled profession, butchering, became a disassembly line job.

The dangerous and inhumane conditions at the Union Stock Yards inspired Upton Sinclair's 1905 classic novel, *The Jungle,* which depicted the daily grind of workers inside the slaughterhouses and packing facilities. So vividly did it describe the widespread filth and disease at the stockyards that the book led to the enactment of the federal Meat Inspection Act of 1906. Sinclair had hoped to touch readers about the wretched treatment of the workers he brought to life in *The Jungle.* But, as he said, "I aimed at the public's heart, and by accident I hit it in the stomach." His description of the doomed pigs seemed to be aimed at both, and affords a glimpse of industrial farming at the beginning:

> It was pork-making by machinery, pork-making by applied mathematics. And yet somehow the most matter of fact person could not help thinking of the hogs; they were so innocent, they came so very trustingly; and they were so very human in their protests— and so perfectly within their rights. They had done nothing to deserve it; and it was adding insult to injury, as the thing was done here, swinging them up in this cold-blooded, impersonal way, without a pretense at apology, without the homage of a tear. Now and then a visitor wept, to be sure; but this slaughtering-machine ran on, visitors or no visitors. It was like some horrible crime committed in a dungeon, all unseen and unheeded, buried out of sight and out of memory.

Accelerating production with methods like these, the five major meat-packing companies had by the second decade of the twentieth century formed the huge Beef Trust. It dominated the means of production and colluded in fixing prices so that ranchers raising beef cattle received very little for their animals. Presented with these abuses, the Federal Trade Commission broke up the trust in 1920, and in 1921 the Packers and Stockyards Administration (P&SA) was created to prevent unfair practices in the industry. Even as the beef industry consolidated and adopted factory-style production methods, up until the late 1930s, most of American agriculture remained much as it had for many decades. Farmers used a mixed crop system, not only producing grains and vegetables for sale in their communities or to local markets but also allowing their cattle and horses, who were used for transportation and to work the land, to obtain much of their own food by grazing. The ranging animals naturally spread their manure, helping to fertilize the fields.

It was during the period after World War II that U.S. agriculture changed almost beyond recognition. When the war ended, both government and industry sought to turn the technology developed for military purposes to civilian uses. This could be described idealistically as turning swords into plowshares, or cynically as looking to expand markets and global influence. One postwar innovation in chemistry was chemical fertilizer, which made it no longer necessary or profitable to use animal manure on crops. Tractors were already replacing workhorses, and livestock and poultry were moved indoors, where they could be raised intensively in controlled conditions (and the weather would have far less influence over production). Crop farmers dedicated themselves to raising ever larger fields of a few, fast-growing varieties of corn and soybeans, much of which was fed to the animals confined inside. Yields, of both animals and crops, increased significantly.

In the 1950s, the call went out from Ezra Taft Benson, secretary of agriculture under President Eisenhower, that farmers had to "get big or get out." Government planners and those involved in the business of agriculture assumed that bigger farms were both more efficient and more productive. For the next fifty-plus years their vision became the dominant reality. In 1950 the United States had 3 million pig farms and 55 million pigs. That's an average of nineteen animals per farm. By 2005, the number of pig-producing farms had dropped to 67,000, less than 3 percent of what existed in 1950. These farms housed 60 million pigs, with some massive industrial production facilities confining many thousands. Over the same period, the number of farms or ranches with beef cattle fell from 4 million to less than 1 million, even as the number of cattle in the United States rose from 77 million to 95 million. Also over the past half century, the number of dairy farms has dropped substantially, from

3.6 million to 78,000, along with the number of dairy cows—from 21 million to 9 million. But because each cow is being pushed harder, we are producing more milk today than fifty years ago.

With chickens the numbers are even more dramatic. The poultry industry was first consolidated on farms in three states, Delaware, Maryland, and Virginia (an area referred to as Delmarva), immediately before and after World War II, and it has been, in sheer volume, the most intensive segment of animal agriculture. In 1950, 50,000 farms produced 630 million meat chickens. That's an average of 12,630 birds per farm. By 2005, the United States had 20,000 fewer farms, but the average number of birds per farm had risen to nearly 300,000, for an astonishing total of 8.7 billion meat chickens. The increase is in part due to consumer trends— Americans simply began eating more chicken, and fast-food chains, recognizing the shift, began to promote chicken products on their menus. Since 1959, the number of egg farms has declined from over 800,000 to less than 100,000 in 2005, while the number of egg-laying hens has fallen to around 340 million from more than 450 million. Like dairy cows, layer hens are vastly more productive than their forebears, together pumping out an extraordinary 90 *billion* eggs in 2005.

Along with the increase in volume and the concentration of animals, the value of each one has declined, another outcome of the economics of supply and demand. If a farmer has, say, thousands of pigs in a shed, he can afford and even expects to lose a certain percentage to injury, illness, or the stresses of overproduction. As long as he maintains his profit margins, the farmer can dismiss the loss as the cost of doing business. As the number of farms has shrunk, so has the number of farmers. In the late nineteenth century, one in four people in the United States lived on a farm. Now it's estimated that only 0.7 percent of the U.S. population are full-time farmers, although many more are involved in the food processing and distribution industry, whose products we see arranged on our supermarket shelves, and whose multimillion-dollar advertising campaigns persuade us to buy and consume those products.

As the animals vanished from the land, the feedlots, slaughterhouses, and factory farms also retreated from view. Chicago's Union Stock Yards has closed, and the facilities of the meat and dairy industry are now mainly seen, smelled, and staffed by the poorest or most unfortunate among us in rural parts of the United States. As in many other sectors of American business, agriculture has come to be defined by huge corporations as smaller producers have been squeezed out. One of the agribusiness giants, ConAgra, produces Armour products, Butterball turkeys, Country Pride, Egg Beaters, Texas BBQ, Swift Premium, and other branded animal products. In 2005, it reported revenues of more than $14 billion and 38,000 employees in more than 130 manufacturing facilities throughout the United States (along with more than twenty plants around the world). Another, Smithfield, grossed $11.84 billion in 2005 and has 50,000 employees in more than forty slaughterhouses and production facilities in the United States and worldwide. Biggest of all are Arkansas-based Tyson, which owns IBP, Madison Foods, and Tyson Poultry, among other brands, and in 2005 had revenues of $26.02 billion and 114,000 employees, and Cargill, whose brands Excel Fresh Meats, Angus Pride, Shady Brook Farms, and Tender Choice, among others, bring in an extraordinary $71 billion a year. As they have expanded in size, these corporations have increased their power in the marketplace. For example, the top four cattle processors, IBP, Monfort (owned by ConAgra), Excel (owned by Cargill), and Farmland National, together control about 80 percent of the market.

Guided by the sternest laws of supply and demand, and protected by immense political influence, factory farming is now the norm, and few working in the industry today can recall a time when things were different. The amount of animal protein produced and consumed in the United States has skyrocketed. In 1950, just over 1 billion farmed animals were killed for food in the United States. By 1975, that number exceeded 3 billion, and in the late 1980s it was more than 6 billion. By 2005 the number neared 10 billion. Along with almost 9 billion chickens, this includes 100 million pigs, 35 million cows and calves, and more than 250 million turkeys.

The Education of a Young Activist

In the 1970s and early 1980s, I knew very little about the vast reach of factory farming and how it was in the process of completely transforming the culture of farming and food in the United States. My mother encouraged me and my siblings to work in the film and television industry to earn college money, and ironically, I ended up in commercials for McDonald's and other fast-food restaurants. Yet I was increasingly impatient and uneasy with what was happening. I began to question some basic assumptions about how I lived and how my actions affected others. And in this, of course, I was not alone.

As a teenager, I hung out on the hillside surrounding the Greek Theater below the Griffith Observatory in the Hollywood hills and listened to the musicians, many of whom were peace activists opposed to America's involvement in the Vietnam War. Peter, Paul and Mary, Joan Baez, Pete Seeger, and others passed through the Greek Theater, and they left their mark on me.

In the late seventies and early eighties, I took an active interest in the conflicts in Latin America and became familiar with the teachings of liberation theology, which—at its best—stood for the idea that the message of the gospels was one of solidarity with the poor and suffering. We're called to answer their need in this life, in the here and now. While I valued what I had learned at Catholic school—and especially Catholicism's basic moral teachings about the strong protecting the weak, and doing unto others as you would have them do unto you—it was hard to avoid noticing a disconnect between what was taught and what was practiced. One had only to walk the streets of downtown Los Angeles to see homeless people wandering about and animals astray and forgotten. Of course, adolescence is a time of idealism, and it's not uncommon for a teenager to believe they're the first to see such wrongs or care about them. It's easy to fault others for not doing their best. But you learn after a while to be more measured in your judgments, more charitable in assessing the motives and efforts of others. And if you look closely enough, wherever there is great need—human or animal—there are always good people rising to answer it.

The most important thing of all, in any case, is to recognize that you can't control others, only yourself. You can be a demanding judge of your own behavior, and I was. I began to ask myself what I was contributing to make the world a kinder place. I did not want to march blindly along, get the right degrees, take the right job, and take my assigned place as a cog in the system. I could not ignore the problems around me.

Throughout high school and college, I looked for ways to make a difference—for instance, by volunteering to spend time with hospitalized children. Even here, however, I felt that everything was too technical, sterile, and inhuman. Adding plants or animals would have improved the atmosphere in the hospital and the quality of the patients' lives. I am pleased that today there is a growing awareness of how animals help people heal, and animal-assisted therapy programs are on the rise. One of my colleagues at Farm Sanctuary and her dog are involved in this kind of work.

I graduated from Loyola High School in 1980, and in those days eighteen-year-old men had to register for the draft. It was a big decision for me, and in the end I registered as a conscientious objector. A year previously, the movie *Hair* had been released, and I was inspired by its story of a farm boy drafted into the Vietnam War who meets up with a group of flower children in New York City. During my senior year, my class staged *Hair* and a lot of my friends were in it.

After graduation, I attended Los Angeles Valley College, a community college in the San Fernando Valley. I took an environmental class there in which I first learned about how quickly the human population was growing and the stresses we were putting on the earth. I later enrolled at California State University, Northridge, and majored in sociology. Soon, though, I found myself wanting to get out and explore the world beyond Los Angeles. So in 1984 I enrolled in a one-year exchange program at the University of Rhode Island. On the East Coast, I loved seeing older buildings and communities—such a contrast from suburban Southern California.

It was at the University of Rhode Island that I heard several people speak who made an impact on me, including the 1960s counterculture activists Jerry Rubin and Abbie Hoffman. In the early 1980s, Rubin had joined "the system," as mainstream society was often referred to then, while Hoffman remained staunchly anti-establishment, and they were staging debates about their different approaches. I also attended a talk by Ralph Nader, the consumer advocate, who at that time was best known for his campaign for automobile safety. He told the students that while we Americans had learned to produce things and were experts at marketing and selling them, we had not really learned how to be responsible consumers. He recalled how resistant the automobile industry had been to making their vehicles safer because, the industry claimed, the changes would compromise the design. He said that "we sacrifice engineering integrity for stylistic pornography," and that concept stuck with me. I thought he was right: we do, all too often, accept something—whether it's a product, a piece of information, or food—because it taps into superficial desires or familiar habits and assumptions that are neither healthy, smart, nor in our or others' best interests.

During the second semester of my program, I moved to Washington, D.C., where I worked as an intern at one of the organizations Nader founded, the U.S. Public Interest Research Group (USPIRG). It was during my time in D.C. that I attended a talk by the astronomer Carl Sagan, who was then renowned for his public television series *Cosmos*. Carl's passion for his subject attracted a huge viewing audience. Sagan told the assembly how *Homo sapiens sapiens* (us) is just one of many millions of species, that we are all "star stuff," and that no species is guaranteed its tenure on the planet. Just as Copernicus and Galileo had discovered that the earth was not the center of the universe, we humans, Sagan said, needed to realize that not everything revolved around us. Sagan was asking us to recognize that we were *part of* our environment rather than *apart from* it, and that if we weren't careful, the consequences of our shortsighted, species-centric actions would be catastrophic for many species, including our own. We were, he said, unraveling the very web of life itself. While our intelligence allowed us to solve problems, we'd created many of those problems for ourselves, and sometimes our "solutions" simply created more difficulties.

During my year away from L.A. and through the summer of 1985, I hitchhiked around the country, trying to keep an open mind and looking for a way of life that would match my values. I traveled from New England to Disney World and Key West, from North Carolina to upstate New York. It was while I was sitting in the back of a pickup truck on my way from Albany to Buffalo, New York, that I first noticed the beauty of upstate New York. Even then I had a feeling about it. The area where I found myself is called the Burned-Over District, a region where many individuals over the years have gone to experience a different form of community or even a kind of enlightenment. Abolitionists such as Harriet Tubman settled there, and the U.S. women's rights movement was born in the district in the nineteenth century. It was home to the Oneida Community, a communalist group that was established in 1848 and closed some years later with mixed results. Many Amish also had settled there. So it's fitting that this part of the world later became home to Farm Sanctuary.

As I traveled and met different people, the subject of factory farming came up again and again. I had first heard serious talk about it at USPIRG, and from friends who had read Frances Moore Lappé's groundbreaking book, *Diet for a Small Planet.* What she documented was new to me. I learned how wasteful factory farming was, how many resources were used to produce meat. Having grain that could be used to feed the world's hungry people fed instead to farm animals struck me as transparently wrong and unjust. I began thinking more seriously about farming—about how we produce our food and how fundamental food is to our existence. It was during that summer that I worked at Greenpeace in Chicago, where I met Lorri, whom I later married and started Farm Sanctuary with, and became a vegetarian. (Some years later, with many shared achievements to remember, Lorri and I went our separate ways.)

The Amish intrigued me in those years, and I found myself trying to understand them. Amish life is defined by values deeper than simply the acquisition of material goods. The goal is to live with integrity, connected to the community and to the earth. I had learned about the Amish in my college sociology classes and how they were known as the "gentle people." Like me, they were opposed to war and violence, and since I was also interested in farming and farm culture (perhaps as a result of my farming ancestors), it seemed to me I needed to pay them a call. So I traveled to Lancaster County in Pennsylvania Dutch country, which, like upstate New York, was home to a large Amish community. I ended up staying in a hotel across the street from the New Holland stockyard, where cows, sheep, and other farm animals were sold. Everyone I met in town seemed to be very proud of it. "This is a historic livestock market," they told me. "It's really interesting. You should see it."

I passed on the invitation at the time, and at the end of that summer I hitchhiked back to California and finished up my sociology degree. But I remembered Lancaster County and the farming it was home to. What I didn't know then was that I would return to the town of Lancaster one year later and meet a sheep who would change my life forever.

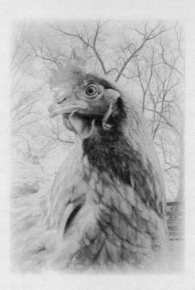

Marmalade

PROFILE: MARMALADE

Marmalade is a small bird with a big personality who makes her presence felt around the Watkins Glen farm. She's curious and very gregarious with other hens, roosters, and people. In fact, she wants to know everything her human caretakers are doing. Even before you enter the yard and barn, Marmalade is at the gate and follows you as you check each bird's health, give them food and water, and move their small wooden enclosures so they can get at the worms and grubs they love underneath the soil.

Marmalade got her name from the color of her feathers, tawny orange with flecks of white, common to the Rhode Island Red breed. When she arrived at Farm Sanctuary, Marmalade was in bad shape, suffering from pneumonia and a condition called air sacculitis, and she could hardly breathe. Her face was swollen and her eyes weren't even visible. When you touched her she screamed, because she couldn't see anything.

The conditions Marmalade had been living in were shocking. On a property in the upstate New York town of Prattsburgh, SPCA officers found dozens of sick, injured, and emaciated animals, all outdoors and none with shelter. Many others had already died. All the survivors were malnourished and suffering from exposure (temperatures in upstate New York can get very cold in the winter). The SPCA took in thirty chickens, mainly roosters, a guinea fowl, and a duck, and called Farm Sanctuary. We agreed to take them all. We were worried that neither Marmalade nor many of the other birds rescued with her would survive. None of them had been cared for adequately, and many of the roosters had severe frostbite.

Once Marmalade and the others arrived at Farm Sanctuary, we kept them all inside so they could stay warm as we nursed them. We gave her and the other birds numerous treatments with antibiotics and provided round-the-clock care. Sadly, we lost one rooster, but the rest made it. Like Marmalade, all the birds from that farm are very sweet-natured. When you help sick animals, they seem to understand. They're grateful, and they don't forgot.

Marmalade remembers the people who nursed her during her recovery, and she shows it every day. Chickens can be extremely friendly and social. In a large flock they are not as interested in people, but in smaller groups the hens and roosters can get very close to you because they get to see you one-on-one, and will often follow you around. Marmalade lives happily with several other hens who were rescued with her as well as a rooster, all of whom got together and formed a flock. The rest of the Prattsburgh roosters share their own private bachelor pad.

CHAPTER TWO

Saving Hilda

Near the end of my last year of college I bought a used 1977 Volkswagen Westphalia van with a pop-top for $3,700. It had a bed on top, another pullout bed on the bottom, a small refrigerator (which never worked very well), a stove powered by a propane tank, and a tiny sink. At the end of the year, Lorri came out to Los Angeles, and in January 1986, the two of us drove across the country to Washington, D.C., to work in the animal advocacy movement.

We were young, fired up, and ready to take on the world. We wanted to make the cruelties of factory farming and its dangers to human health and the environment better known to the public. We also got involved in other aspects of the animal rights movement. That winter, four of us living in D.C. decided to attend an anti-fur demonstration at Macy's, which then sold and continues to sell fur. The protest was organized by a very active group in New York City, Trans-Species Unlimited, which held a number of highly visible and successful animal rights protests in the mid- to late 1980s.

On the four-hour drive up to New York, we began batting around ideas for other ways of documenting and letting the public know about what life was like for the billions of animals caught up in the industrialized farm system in the United States. We agreed we could reach many more people if we got on the road than we could from our office in Washington, D.C. By the end of the trip, Lorri and I had settled on a plan to start Farm Sanctuary. No one had a clear idea of what it was going to be, except that somehow it would combat factory farming and do so through some form of education and outreach. Back then, we didn't know what we'd be doing in the next five hours, never mind the next five years. We hit on a word that resonated with all of us—*sanctuary*—though we really had no clear idea that we would create an actual farm that would rescue farmed animals, take care of them, and encourage people to visit. We simply latched on to the idea of an oasis and decided to see where it led.

One of our fellow activists was so enthusiastic about the idea that he told us we could live and work in a row house he owned at 224 Stroud Street in the Browntown area of Wilmington, Delaware. Rent-free and available sounded good to us, so a couple of weeks later we left D.C. and moved in to begin Farm Sanctuary—whatever that meant. The house was not luxurious. In fact, it was a mess (read: close to uninhabitable). The previous tenant had died suddenly and unexpectedly, and the house had quickly fallen into disrepair. The water pipes leaked into the kitchen ceiling, which eventually collapsed, and that was just the start of a long list of needed repairs. For the next few months we had our work cut out for us.

In April 1986, Farm Sanctuary was incorporated and we began producing advocacy literature. We knew, generally speaking, the conditions for animals on factory farms and in slaughterhouses, but little about the specifics and had never visited a factory farm. We felt that in order to be credible advocates we should have firsthand knowledge. Despite the publication in 1980 of *Animal Factories,* Jim Mason and Peter Singer's seminal work, relatively little documentation was publicly available on American industrialized animal agriculture.

Life Inside the Stockyards

It was the historian and activist Bernard Unti, then working at the American Anti-Vivisection Society, who first suggested we investigate the conditions at the stockyard in nearby Lancaster, Pennsylvania. I would soon confront the sights, smells, and otherworldly sounds of the modern livestock trade.

Lancaster Stockyards was one of the oldest in the United States, incorporated in 1895. By 1908, the stockyard was dealing with 170,000 cattle a year and still growing. At its peak in the 1940s, 450,000 animals a year were brought to market there. It was at Lancaster that livestock was sold and then slaughtered for meat for the growing populations of cities such as Baltimore and Philadelphia. Lancaster was known as a terminal market, similar to the Union Stock Yards in Chicago and the South St. Paul Stockyards in Minnesota—and as the name suggests, a terminal market is the last stop for an animal before he or she is killed.

When we first visited in the mid-1980s, Lancaster was still handling over 300,000 animals a year from as far away as Montana and Texas, but it was no longer the economic powerhouse it once had been. Increasingly, it was serving niche markets, such as sheep and goat meat for ethnic communities on the East Coast, as well as marketing animals from Amish and Mennonite farms in the region. Both the Amish and Mennonites, who prided themselves on their resistance to the mores of American industrial society, were accommodating themselves to the modern world. Some were driving motorized vehicles rather than horse-drawn buggies, including the "black bumper Mennonites," who'd painted their cars' chrome bumpers black so they wouldn't appear too ostentatious. Because the law required that milk be refrigerated, many of the farmers had begun using electricity. And since banks tended to provide loans only if you adopted the latest technology and intensified operations, Amish and Mennonite farmers were beginning to practice aspects of factory farming, such as confining their hens in small "battery" cages and male calves in tiny crates to produce veal.

Lancaster Stockyards was huge, stretching across twenty-two acres to the north of the town. It was shaped like a grid and consisted of outdoor wooden pens with large gates, "long-legged barns" for the adult cattle, and "short-legged barns" for calves, pigs, sheep, and goats. These areas were bisected with alleyways, loading docks, and auction rings, where animals were paraded and then sold to the highest bidder. Trucks would travel from farms to the stockyard and back up to the loading dock, which was usually about four or so feet off the ground, and the animals would be herded down a ramp and through the alleyways into the holding pens.

Much of the stockyard was paved with cobblestones, which a stockyard worker once told me had been brought to America as ballast in empty ships that sailed from Europe. These ships would then return heavy with food and other products from the New World. I spent countless hours walking on those cobblestones and through the alleyways that connected the pens with the auction rings.

Lancaster was the first stockyard I ever visited, and over the spring and summer of 1986, I went there often. It was completely different from anything I'd experienced before. The smells of manure and death were everywhere. On sale days the market bustled—sheep and goats bleated, cows mooed, truck engines rumbled as they backed up to the loading dock, and ramps clanked as they were put into place. You could hear banging as the animals shifted their weight inside the trucks and as their hoofs struck the hard metal floors. And always there was the squealing of pigs. The very buildings of Lancaster Stockyards seemed to groan. Because the wooden corrals were covered in sheet metal, which expanded and contracted in the heat and cold, the roofs creaked constantly. In summer the stockyard was wretchedly humid; in winter everything, including the water in the troughs for the animals, froze.

I quickly found there was little room for sentimentality inside the stockyard. Men yelled at the animals as they herded them through the alleyways, hitting them with whips and canes and shocking them with electric prods to get them to move as quickly as possible to their pens or the auction ring. The animals looked terrified and often scrambled over each other to avoid being hit. During our earliest visits we spent most of our time taking photographs and then, later, shooting video footage. We also kept a lookout for stockyard workers and tried to avoid trouble, but because the stockyard was a public market, it was hard for its management to deny us the right to be there.

Almost as soon as we began to visit Lancaster Stockyards, we would come across animals lying dead or injured in the alleyways or the holding pens. Either they had been hurt in the stockyard during handling or unloading, or they had arrived injured or sick and were unable to stand. Those who were dead on arrival or who'd died soon after were picked up and moved to what was unsentimentally called the dead pile. At Lancaster, the dead pile was a concrete slab with cinder-block walls on three sides located at the back of one of the buildings near the railroad tracks. (Trains had been the main method of transporting animals to the stockyard until the 1960s, when trucks became the sole form of delivery.)

The carcasses on the dead pile would stay there until the renderer came around. Depending on the level of the animals' decay, the renderer would skin the bodies of their hides for leather, boil them and siphon off the fat for soap, or use the flesh to feed other animals. The rest would be turned into fertilizer. Disposing of dead or dying animals at the dead pile was a service the stockyard provided to farmers, and it saved the renderer from making trips to individual farms to gather up the bodies.

One hot and humid Sunday in August 1986, as we walked by the dead pile, we saw carcasses of a cow, a couple of pigs, and some sheep decaying in the heat—nothing unusual. The body of a calf had decomposed enough for us to see his rib cage. The stench was overpowering. A swarm of thick, fat maggots, inches deep, was burrowing into the calf's flesh, buzzing as they did so. To the side of the pile near one of the walls, we saw a sheep lying on her side. As we approached, something remarkable happened: the sheep lifted up her head and looked at us.

I was stunned. Lorri and I looked at each other in horror. Without exchanging a word we both knew that we couldn't let the animal stay where she was. Our first, overpowering thought was that somehow we had to get this sheep out of there.

Technically, though, we did not own the sheep and therefore had no right to remove her. We were in no state of mind to ask for permission to take the sheep, and it was Sunday, so there was no one around to ask even if we'd thought to do so. Industrial stockyards such as Lancaster are often very big. While a worker called a checker might be at the front gate twenty-four hours a day to account for animals when they arrived and were shipped out, we often walked the property without seeing any staff. Besides, we were in a part of the stockyard that no one had any interest in investigating. We were essentially picking through trash.

Because of where we'd found her and the state she was in, we had little hope that the sheep would survive. She likely would need to be euthanized. But we knew we couldn't leave her on the dead pile to linger, possibly for days. We got the van, lifted her into the space behind the front seats, and started driving around town, looking for a veterinarian to treat her. We didn't stop to think about what we were doing. We just knew it had to be done.

Finally we found one. The vet came out to the van and started palpating the sheep's body. The sheep, who was about six months old, barely more than a lamb, started showing signs of life. She began to breathe more easily and move. Even though she remained remarkably quiet, within twenty minutes she was standing up, right there in the van. Far from needing to be euthanized, the sheep was on her way to a full recovery. We took the sheep, whom we named Hilda after Farm Sanctuary's first volunteer intern, back to the house in Wilmington, placed her in a little shed in our backyard, gave her water and food, shade and care, and she recovered quickly. A day or so later we had her shorn of her coat, which was uncomfortable in the summer heat.

Our decision to take Hilda had been immediate. This was the first time we'd come across a live animal on the stockyard's dead pile, and we were stunned that there was a living, breathing, feeling being amid the rotting remains. What callousness, what carelessness and disrespect for a live animal, to write her off as dead and throw her away like garbage! We were there to affirm that she was *not* garbage—she was a living creature, and she deserved better than this.

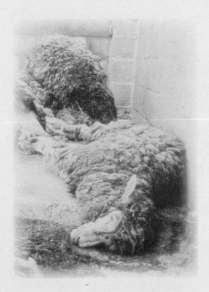
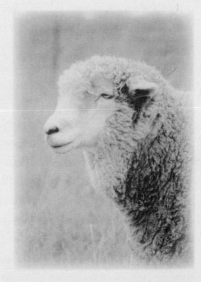

Hilda at the stockyards   *Hilda at Farm Sanctuary*

After Hilda's rescue, we pieced together how she could have ended up where she did. Most likely Hilda had been packed into a standard livestock truck coming from a farm in New York along with hundreds of other sheep and inadequate ventilation. She had probably collapsed from heat exhaustion during the long journey before she reached the stockyard. It seemed obvious she'd been on the floor of the truck for some time, since her full wool coat was caked with excrement, most likely from other sheep. When the truck arrived at Lancaster Stockyards, the sheep who'd survived the trip had walked off, but several, including Hilda, were motionless and presumed dead. So all of them were dumped on the dead pile. Hilda was the lone survivor. She was lucky in other ways, too. It had rained the previous day, and that perhaps had cooled her down and given her a little water to drink so she didn't die of thirst. Hilda was also slightly to the side of the pile rather than on the top or, worse, at the bottom, where she could have suffocated. This had left her relatively free of maggots.

We informed the local humane society about what had happened to Hilda to see if they would prosecute, assuming there was a legal statute that applied to this situation. Their reply shocked us. They told us they wouldn't pursue the case. Indeed, they appeared indifferent and were uninterested in prosecuting those responsible for discarding Hilda. Still, we pushed for an investigation and discovered the identity of the trucker. Regarding who "owned" her: all the evidence pointed to the president of the stockyards himself, Bill McCoy. When we asked the humane society to look at the case again in light of this new information, they replied that the trucker had said he was sorry for what had happened to Hilda and that we shouldn't take the issue any further—they certainly didn't plan to.

But an apology didn't seem like enough. Here was a clear case of neglect and liability. Perhaps I was naive, but I was surprised, first that such a thing could happen and, second, that those charged with preventing cruelty to animals would do nothing about it. We felt we had a responsibility to pursue the matter since those who should have been looking out for the animals' welfare wouldn't. We had no interest in a vendetta against the person who'd abandoned Hilda for dead, but somebody or something had to be made accountable so that it wouldn't happen again.

To our dismay, we discovered that it wasn't entirely clear there *was* anything illegal about what had taken place. In Pennsylvania, normal agricultural operations are exempted from state prosecution, and as we were to find out many times in the coming years, sick and dying animals in stockyards were all too "normal." In fact, it was we who were at risk of prosecution! Because Hilda had recovered and stood up, she became valuable again and suitable for slaughter. We could have been charged with property theft.

Downers

The decision to help that first animal in need was momentous. Hilda became a symbol of the larger problem of indifference to farmed animals in general and sick animals in particular, and it was her rescue that launched Farm Sanctuary's first major advocacy effort. Hilda made us into an organization—as well as an actual, physical sanctuary.

Factory farms and stockyards have words to describe animals in Hilda's condition: they are called downed animals or downers. Although the terms have come into more general use in the last few years, particularly because of the emergence of mad cow disease, in those days the terms were used only by the industry and referred to animals down on the ground, unable to move on their own because they were sick, injured, or dying.

It wasn't long before we found other downed animals at Lancaster in the alleyways and pens. We had identified a clear problem—incapacitated animals left to suffer with no treatment or care. It was a problem with a clear solution—a no-downer policy, whereby downed animals would not be sold through the stockyard. If farmers had to take responsibility for the cost of providing veterinary care or humanely euthanizing downed animals, rather than being financially rewarded for selling them, we believed their behavior would change. We hoped they would treat their animals better before sending them to slaughter to keep them from becoming downed in the first place, or insist on better conditions during transport to slaughterhouses. With this as our objective, we initiated the no-downer campaign at Lancaster Stockyards.

I made it clear to Bill McCoy, the stockyard's president, that ultimately he had to take responsibility for the animals in the stockyard's custody. It was in the stockyard's best interest, I argued, to care for the animals or euthanize them, because it meant that healthier animals were going to go into the food chain, lessening the risk of disease. We'd also discovered that it's impossible to move large downed animals compassionately. They are often dragged with chains or pushed with tractors and forklifts. I have documented many instances of this, and it's always heartbreaking. It also takes considerable time and labor. Clearly, it was preferable for the stockyard, and the animals, to put downers out of their misery quickly.

The stockyard was cautious in its response. Company officials told us they agreed with our position that downed animals should not be marketed, but were reluctant to institute a no-downer policy because other stockyards—like the one nearby in New Holland—were selling downed animals who arrived on the premises still alive, and if Lancaster didn't also, it would lose that business. Since the stockyard refused to take concrete action, we continued documenting the inhumane conditions inside the facility and then shared it with the public, media, and other activists. In 1987 and 1988 we organized public meetings that brought further media and community attention to the issue of downers at Lancaster Stockyards and brought us volunteers who went into the stockyard to both document and rescue downed animals.

It came as no surprise to me that the abuse of downed animals sparked outrage in the community. Even though we were in the middle of farm country and were ruffling the industry's feathers, people could see that there was something fundamentally wrong in how sick or injured "food" animals were being treated.

At times, the atmosphere could get pretty heated. The workers, as well as McCoy, were very resistant to any change in the way things were done. Their attitude was that they'd been running a stockyard for nearly a century, they knew what they were doing, and nobody had any right to question them. On one occasion, I was at the stockyard with a local newspaper reporter, talking about the downed animal issue, when we saw a downed pig near the unloading dock. At that point, Bill McCoy showed up and we had a tense exchange that almost came to blows. That afternoon, though, McCoy did the right thing and agreed to allow the suffering animal to be euthanized.

Even though Lancaster's officials initially dismissed our concerns about animal welfare, we continued to pursue the matter and eventually reached an agreement. The stockyard would call us when sick or dying animals arrived at the facility, and we would provide them with veterinary care or, if the situation was hopeless, humane euthanasia. In practice, however, we didn't receive any calls, so we began to visit the stockyard again. Not surprisingly, nothing had really changed, and we found more downed animals. After more efforts on our behalf to raise public awareness, McCoy eventually assured us that he would honor our agreement, and we *did* begin receiving calls. Over the next several months, we made numerous trips to Lancaster Stockyards to rescue downed animals or have those who could not be saved euthanized.

We had made our offer to the stockyard to care for downed animals on the understanding that it would be an interim measure, but the stockyard seemed to be making no real effort to develop a longer-term policy. In fact, I believe that in a calculated ploy, they tried to overwhelm us emotionally, logistically, and financially to crush our spirits. They called us to come to the stockyard repeatedly to euthanize suffering animals. Perhaps they wanted us to feel that the task was too enormous to make any difference. Maybe they wanted to close us down before, as they feared, we could find a way to close down the stockyard—something we weren't even thinking about. While we could perhaps dream that the animals' suffering at the stockyard would end, the day-to-day rescue efforts were all we could handle. Farm Sanctuary then was still a very new, all-volunteer organization, with limited funds, and calling vets to euthanize the animals was not cheap.

The stockyard's cynicism was made clear to me one day when I got a call that more than twenty pigs needed to be euthanized. Such a large number of downed animals at one time was very unusual. When I arrived at the stockyard with the veterinarian, I had to hold the pigs, one by one, as the vet administered lethal injections. It was one of the most difficult and painful things I've ever had to do. I later heard that the stockyard management had told farmers to bring in their "junk" so that we would have to deal with it. Apparently they hoped to break our will. Ironically, the effort had only confirmed what we were saying: that the stockyard was serving as a dumping ground for sick animals who shouldn't have been entering the food chain anyway.

When I reiterated to McCoy that it was the stockyard and not we who had the responsibility for the downed animals, he replied, "I put the monkey on your back."

"Bill," I reminded him firmly, "it's *your* monkey." This episode gave me one of the first inklings of the problem of passing the buck in order to save a buck—a problem that affects the entire farmed animal industry. Farmers were unwilling to deal with their sick animals, so they dumped them at the stockyard, making it the stockyard's problem. Meanwhile, the stockyard wanted to make the sick animals *our* problem. It seemed we were the only ones unwilling to pass on our own costs and liability.

We worked to bring the issue into the spotlight and took immediate action to save animals when we could, but there was no question that the responsibility for solving the larger problem lay squarely with the industry. On Memorial Day 1988 we staged our first and only rally outside Lancaster Stockyards. More than five hundred people from all over the mid-Atlantic region, as well as Lancaster itself, joined us to call for better treatment of animals in the food system. We had a series of speakers, including factory farming expert Jim Mason, whose support gave momentum to the cause and our fledgling organization. The demonstration also caught the attention of the print and broadcast press.

The stockyard realized its position was becoming untenable, even though it continued to misbehave. In one instance, a sheep who had been left on the dead pile was actually brought back into the stockyard so he couldn't be rescued or otherwise cared for. But in June 1988 the stockyard started shouldering some of the burden—it acquired a captive bolt gun, which kills animals by driving a metal rod into their brain, so that downed animals could be euthanized on the spot. The captive bolt gun or another firearm is a common method of euthanasia in the farming industry, despite problems with their effectiveness. Later that year Lancaster Stockyards announced that it would no longer accept downed animals. We celebrated: it was a major victory, and our first one.

An Impasse

My philosophy of activism has been guided by the late animal rights and labor activist Henry Spira. He understood the importance of being reasonable and giving your opponent the opportunity to do the right thing. Spira believed you should be respectful but firm and clear in your dealings with opponents. Our no-downer campaign followed Spira's example in giving the stockyard an opportunity to engage with us. When it didn't respond to our private overtures, we contacted the media and held public meetings and a demonstration. When the stockyard initiated a no-downer policy, we praised and thanked it. But we also remained skeptical and vigilant.

Sadly, despite the stockyard's assurances that it had changed course, over the following years we found that downed animals were still being left to suffer and die at Lancaster Stockyards. We appealed repeatedly to local law enforcement officers about this, but they remained indifferent. Frustrated by the legal authorities' failure to address downed animal abuse at the stockyard, in 1991 Farm Sanctuary formally incorporated in Pennsylvania as a Society for the Prevention of Cruelty to Animals (SPCA). Since the stockyard wasn't enforcing its own policy, we were once more required to act ourselves, and as an SPCA we could authorize our representative to enforce Pennsylvania's anti-cruelty laws.

We appointed Keith Mohler, who came from the surrounding community and had been volunteering with Farm Sanctuary to monitor stockyard conditions, as our first humane officer. On July 22, 1992, during a visit to the stockyard, Keith came across two cows in a pen who were clearly very sick but still standing. He asked stockyard workers if the cows were receiving veterinary care and was told that they were about to be picked up and taken to slaughter. Since they were not technically downed, Keith couldn't take any action. He had to take the workers at their word. But when he returned the following day, Keith found that while one of the cows was gone, the other, now too sick even to stand, was still in the pen.

"You said this was going to be taken care of. What's going on here?" Keith asked the stockyard attendant, who replied that the remaining cow was "written off as dead." Despite repeated requests and calls to the stockyard's management, no one would provide veterinary care or euthanize the cow. We learned that the animal had been purchased, and therefore was owned, by a slaughterhouse in North Carolina. When the slaughterhouse's trucker came to the stockyard, he had chosen to leave the cow in the pen because she couldn't walk onto his truck. Perhaps he hoped to sell her later to a local downed-animal dealer so she could be slaughtered for food.

Eventually, at around ten o'clock in the evening, in the absence of appropriate action on the part of the stockyard, Keith called a veterinarian, Dr. Barry Harris, to examine the cow. "When I arrived," Dr. Harris later wrote in a statement, "the cow was in left lateral recumbency and bloated. She had mastitis [an udder infection]. Her legs were in such poor shape that she was unable to rise." The cow was clearly in pain, and Harris elected to put her out of her misery. Soon after, Farm Sanctuary received a bill for $401.50. Since the cow could no longer be slaughtered for human food, the stockyard decided that *we* should pay her market value.

This demonstrated another absurd feature of the economics of farming. Clearly, the humane thing to do was to euthanize the cow. If she'd died without the vet's intervention, insurance probably would have covered her market price; if she'd survived, a local slaughterhouse might have paid something for her meat. Euthanizing her meant a financial loss—it was cheaper to leave the cow alive and suffering. Economic interests were in direct conflict with humane concerns.

Naturally, we were outraged at being billed for doing the decent thing—which was the stockyard's responsibility in the first place. Instead of paying the bill, Keith filed cruelty charges against Lancaster Stockyards for failing to provide the cow with needed food, water, shelter, and veterinary care. "I'm not jubilant about having to file cruelty charges," Keith told a journalist. "It's not a landmark victory but a breakdown in the cooperative system." The farming community began to recognize that it had a problem that stonewalling wouldn't solve. As an opinion piece in *Lancaster Farming* in August 1992 stated: "The moral of the story is this: don't send downed animals to market. Take the loss of one animal at home rather than create a situation that opponents of agriculture can use to destroy the livestock industry."

Lancaster Stockyards, however, didn't take *Lancaster Farming*'s advice. In response to the cruelty charges, an attorney representing the stockyard sent us a letter citing a Pennsylvania legal code that advised us that we were no longer allowed to enter the stockyard premises. If we did, we would be considered trespassers and subject to criminal prosecution. "You have been warned," the letter read. "If you enter the premises of the Lancaster Stockyards, you do so at your peril." I knew we could not take such a notice lightly. (I had heard about property owners shooting trespassers.) McCoy was as emphatic as his lawyer's letter. "We have always operated under the contention that we have nothing to hide," he told a local reporter. "But it's gotten to the point that I don't want them coming in here anymore. They have no right to. It's time to put an end to this."

That we had reached this impasse after Farm Sanctuary had worked for five years with the stockyard, raising public awareness and dealing with downed animals ourselves, was particularly distressing. We had attempted to cooperate with the staff and management of the stockyard. Despite the chronic tension inherent in a relationship between those whose business was commodifying animals and those trying to save them, some downed animals had been treated with a little dignity. But now, Lancaster Stockyards and Farm Sanctuary were on opposite sides of the issue, and a court would determine whether leaving a downed animal to suffer and die was outside the bounds of acceptable conduct under Pennsylvania's anti-cruelty laws.

Court cases rarely run smoothly or according to plan. At the first hearing, our case was dismissed when the stockyard's attorney, whom we learned also represented the local humane enforcement agency and later became Lancaster's mayor, alleged that the complaint didn't accurately identify the specific cow involved. The stockyard supposedly did not know which cow it had allegedly mistreated. It was a strange assertion to make, since the stockyard apparently knew exactly which cow was involved when it arranged to send us a bill for her after she was euthanized!

The dismissal was a setback but not the end of the matter. Keith refiled the charges, this time providing more specific information and noting the exact pen where the downed cow was found. For us, it was an open-and-shut case. The stockyard had unambiguous knowledge of the animal's condition over two days. A veterinarian had examined the animal, clearly said that she was in bad shape, had written down his diagnosis, and had then euthanized her. That Harris, the vet, had taken this action and also provided a statement testifying to this effect was significant and commendable, because veterinarians who deal with animal agriculture are usually reluctant to speak out when the industry for which they do the bulk of their work is under fire.

In spite of various attempts by the stockyard's lawyer to have the case dismissed a second time, the hearing was allowed to go forward and the evidence was presented. Ironically, it was the checker at Lancaster Stockyards, a real character named Billy and something of a local legend, who helped to swing things our way. Billy told the truth about how the downed cow had been written off as dead. On April 27, 1993, Lancaster Stockyards was convicted of denying proper veterinary care to an animal.

We were extremely pleased. The conviction proved that blatant farm animal cruelty is unacceptable, even in farming communities. Although Pennsylvania exempted "normal agricultural operations" from anti-cruelty statutes, the court determined that leaving a downed animal to suffer at a stockyard without providing needed veterinary care was neither normal nor acceptable. It wasn't a huge monetary victory: the conviction required the stockyard to pay a fine of only $150 plus $72 in court costs. But the time and effort we had put in were worth it. It was an important legal victory.

We didn't, though, have much time to savor it. Unfortunately, angered by its conviction, Lancaster Stockyards went on the offensive again. Its attorney asserted that Farm Sanctuary had acted improperly and that the case raised constitutional issues about the actions of animal advocates. "If we decide to make a big deal of this," McCoy told the local newspaper, "we're going to get the whole industry involved, appeal, fight, and win this damn thing, ban these people and get them out of the industry." Agribusiness also viewed the ruling with alarm. Its lobbyists worked with legislators in Harrisburg, Pennsylvania, who had been cultivated through years of campaign contributions and social outings, and a bill was introduced that would have prevented humane enforcement agents from protecting farm animals under Pennsylvania's anti-cruelty laws. So profoundly contradictory and extreme was this legislation that over the next few years, Farm Sanctuary joined with various organizations in Pennsylvania to stop agribusiness from undoing the authority granted under state law for humane law enforcement.

Eventually, a compromise was reached. It preserved humane officers' authority to protect farm animals but set new limitations on enforcement and new requirements for their training. Keith was appointed one of the instructors for the humane officer training. To his chagrin, the teaching venue he was assigned was also used as a university "meat lab" where food animals' bodies are cut into pieces and the cuts then assessed for quality. The point is to teach students what is desirable meat. It was as if the authorities wanted to remind Keith and the others present that farm animals were essentially meat and therefore deserved limited, if any, protection.

An Eventual Victory

Our campaign to make Lancaster Stockyards institute a no-downer policy had far-reaching impact. In 1986, when we began, the stockyard was considered a pillar of the local community and was looking forward to celebrating its hundredth anniversary. We, meanwhile, were outsiders, vegetarian animal rights activists, "absolutely radical," as Bill McCoy called us at one point—which didn't win us many allies in Lancaster. As it turned out, however, the plight of downed animals went from being a marginal issue to a central one within the animal agriculture industry. It even became a national debate. Later, McCoy himself acknowledged that our position was justified: "Our first reaction was, 'Who do they think they are?' We weren't going to cooperate in any way," he told a journalist. "But now I think cooperation is in both our best interests. Our industry, in general, can clean up its act a little."

As the scope of Farm Sanctuary's work was expanding, we still kept tabs on Lancaster Stockyards. By the mid-1990s, it had gone into a steep decline. "Lancaster Stockyards, Once the Largest East of Chicago, Hangs in There," ran the headline of a 1995 article in a Lancaster newspaper. "What do you think of when someone mentions the Lancaster Stockyards?" asked its author, Jack Brubaker. "Do you think of a vibrant livestock trading center, or do you imagine a collection of buildings and animals that are ready to fall down?"

Lancaster was fading along with independent stockyards all over the country. They were being replaced by what are known as "buying stations," run by vertically integrated agribusinesses such as Smithfield. Under these systems, a single corporation does all the purchasing, so it sets the price. Historically, stockyards such as Lancaster formed free markets where animals could be valued by independent buyers bidding on them. No preset price was put on the animals farmers brought to market. Also, unlike stockyards, buying stations aren't a public market. They consist of unloading docks and ramps and pens. The stockyards' auction ring, with its bleachers for buyers to judge the animals, doesn't exist at a buying station. There's no need, since there's only one buyer.

While I am anything but nostalgic for Lancaster's heyday, stockyards were an important part of the farming community. At some of the stockyards I visited over the years, I saw picnic benches or even a restaurant and people telling stories and exchanging ideas about farming practices and other issues of the day. The new system offers none of that. Instead, farmers are individual units competing with each other in an isolated and atomized environment.

In April 2006, almost two decades to the day after Farm Sanctuary was incorporated, Lancaster Stockyards announced that it was closing amid speculation that its twenty-two acres would be sold off for development as stores or offices. Recently, I had the chance to visit Lancaster Stockyards again. I found a very different place than the one I'd known. Instead of slamming gates and screaming workers, quiet had descended. I was struck by the way the old pens and structures were being reclaimed by nature. Trees and vines were taking over buildings, and grass was growing through cracks in the cement. This facility that had been a site of cruel exploitation for decades was being transformed.

I don't mourn the stockyard, but I do wish the land could be used for something other than commercial development. I would love for it to sustain its connection to the local agricultural economy by becoming a farmers' market or even perhaps a vegan organic farm. Better laws and tax incentives could help usher in such a needed transformation in Lancaster and in many other similar places across the rural United States.

A few years ago, I received a Christmas gift from my friends Cayce Mell and Jason Tracy, who used to operate a sanctuary for farmed animals in Pennsylvania. The cardboard package, which was a little less than a foot square, was very heavy, and I wondered what on earth it could contain. When I opened the box, I found a gray rectangular stone with a note that read: "Thought you should have this. It is a small piece of a big part of your history. From the belly of the beast, a cobblestone from Lancaster Stockyards." Next to the Schwinn Sting-Ray I received for Christmas when I was a boy, it was probably one of the most fitting and thoughtful gifts I've ever received.

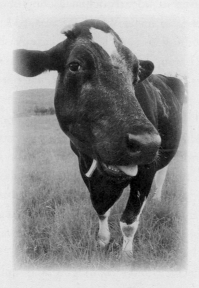

Maya

PROFILE: MAYA

When I first saw Maya, she was a tiny black and white calf, just a few days old, huddled in a corner behind one of the gates at Lancaster Stockyards. She was down and unable to walk through the stockyard. I lifted her out from behind the gate and took her home. When I saw she was limping, I drove her to the New Bolton Veterinary Center, part of the University of Pennsylvania. The young vet on duty said she would try to flush out an infected joint in Maya's front leg. The vet had never done such a procedure before, but I agreed she should go ahead. As Maya recovered I spent a lot of time with her, and her leg healed completely. Maya and I became very close and remained so even as she grew to be a full-grown cow.

One day, a Farm Sanctuary rescue brought in a number of calves from an abusive veal facility. We decided to put them in a pasture with Maya, thinking that she would care for them like an adoptive mother. Maya was always very maternal, even though she never had any calves of her own. As with all calves born to dairy cows, she had been taken from her own mother almost at birth. Maya watched over the calves, protecting and loving them as if they were her own.

Back then, in the 1980s, we didn't know as much about animals' emotions as we do now, and we didn't have the space to keep all the calves. So when adopters offered to take them, we were thrilled. The calves would be able to live the rest of their lives in comfortable places, and room would open up to take in other needy animals. As it happened, we transported the calves to their new homes all in one day. In hindsight, I can see that I made a terrible decision. Suddenly Maya had no calves, and she was bereft and angry. After the calves were removed, she rolled on her back and wailed and could not be consoled.

One day, many years later, I came to visit Maya in the herd at the Watkins Glen shelter. I hadn't seen her for a long time. "Maya," I called to her, as I walked through the pasture. Maya looked at me and began running, not toward me but *at* me, bellowing. In fact, she ran me right off that pasture. I had to jump a fence and lost a shoe in the mud as I ran. I'd been the one who had broken her heart and betrayed her trust, and she hadn't forgotten. I've also thought that Maya's reaction could have stemmed from a feeling that I'd abandoned her. In the early years I spent much of my time on the farm and had lots of direct contact with the animals, including Maya. But as Farm Sanctuary grew, my role and responsibilities changed, and I found myself away from the farm much of the time. Maya might have felt that loss more than I'd ever imagined.

Whatever Maya was expressing that day in the pasture, I learned a lesson in a very direct way: animals have deep emotions, and you cannot assume they aren't forming bonds with other animals or with you. Over the years, as we learned more about the animals' psychology, we instituted a policy that all Farm Sanctuary animals adopted out to new homes have to be placed with at least one companion of their own species.

Happily, in the intervening years, Maya has nurtured many newly rescued calves at Farm Sanctuary, who have gone on to join the herd. But they remain close to Maya and even as adults still look to her for guidance and approval. Maya was the first downed calf I rescued, and she's now over twenty years old: a matriarch and the oldest cow at our Watkins Glen shelter.

CHAPTER THREE

Mad Cows and Washington

By 1991, Farm Sanctuary had grown beyond being just a shelter for rescued farmed animals. We were beginning to have an impact on policies and practices in the animal agriculture industry. We also found ourselves on more solid footing financially than when we had begun in 1986.

Back in those early days, Farm Sanctuary funded itself by selling vegetarian hot dogs at Grateful Dead concerts, an idea that Lorri and I'd had when we attended a Dead concert in San Francisco on New Year's Eve 1986. It was the first time I'd been to see the Grateful Dead, and as we observed the scene, we began to realize that people needed something to eat during the epic shows, and the audience would likely be receptive to a message of peace, love, tofu—and animal rights.

Beginning in 1986, when we were not producing educational literature on factory farming or visiting stockyards and researching the animal agriculture industry, we went on tour with the Grateful Dead, mainly on the East Coast. We had veggie dogs, chili dogs, kraut dogs, and dogs with "the works," which included vegetarian chili and sauerkraut. On a good day we would sell hundreds of vegetarian hot dogs at a single concert. At a dollar a dog (more for the extras), we could earn what (for us) was serious money. We bought the veggie dogs from a center run by Seventh-day Adventists near Washington, D.C. Initially our orders were small, but as we began to sell more dogs we purchased as many as we could stack in the van, and hit the road. We reached critical veggie dog mass on one trip—we were so loaded down the van broke an axle. We also stocked up on Fantastic Foods veggie chili mix in bulk. We bought the rest of our supplies—sauerkraut, pita bread (which we used for the bun), ketchup, and mustard—locally, in the city where the Dead were performing.

The van I'd bought in L.A. became central to all our operations. We rescued Hilda and many others in that van, we slept in it when we traveled with the Dead, and we used it for numerous investigations. When we'd arrive at a concert, we'd set up the propane stove on which we cooked the veggie dogs right in front of the van. We'd also set up a large display of photos and leaflets that showed farmed animals confined in cages or crates, being trucked to slaughter, or with their horns removed or beaks cut back. Those were all standard practices in industrial agriculture then, as they are today. For some concertgoers, the photographic displays were shocking. Many were so moved they broke down in tears.

We toured for a couple of weeks at a time, making a few thousand dollars on each trip. Since Farm Sanctuary was an entirely volunteer organization in those days, it was enough to pay for the production of our literature and our daily expenses. I also supplemented our income teaching basic math and English at a teaching center in downtown Wilmington, Delaware. Neither of us was a true Deadhead, but we enjoyed the whole scene. It was a unique traveling community. Some of the Deadheads were hedonistic and narrow-minded, but others were cause-oriented and had emerged from the same musical culture as Joan Baez and Peter, Paul, and Mary. Many were receptive to our concerns and message of animal rights.

By 1990, we had developed a base of support for Farm Sanctuary's work and no longer had to bankroll our work traveling with the Dead. The faithful green van became a full-time research and rescue vehicle. In 1995, after almost 200,000 miles, many bumps and bruises, and one considerable fender-bender, it was retired. For years, the van sat rusting in the parking lot near the visitors' center in Watkins Glen until the father of one of our staff members kindly sorted out the dents, cleaned it up, and painted the van a bright avocado green to match its original color. At Farm Sanctuary, even old jalopies get a second chance.

Now it sits in one of our storage barns, full of memories, its cabinets and sink still festooned with the bumper stickers from the Grateful

Dead ("No Time to Hate," "Make Tapes, Not War") and our activism ("I Don't Eat My Friends," "Friends Don't Let Friends Eat Meat"). The van wasn't much to look at, but it was sturdy and reliable, and it birthed and carried our mission-driven organization for many years. It reminds me that you can achieve amazing things even by the humblest means.

Finding a Larger Community

As Farm Sanctuary started growing and our goals became bigger, we found that others across the United States were doing similar work. And we started finding ways we could work together to generate change on a larger scale.

From November 1989 to May 1991, an activist named Becky San-stedt regularly visited a stockyard in South St. Paul, Minnesota, and filmed what she saw. At that time the stockyard was the second largest in the country and belonged to the United Stockyards Corporation, owner of seven of the largest stockyards in the United States. Her forty-four hours of video footage documented conditions at the stockyard that were nothing less than appalling. Her tapes captured pigs with volleyball-sized tumors and "cancer eye cows," cows whose eye sockets were infected and infested with flies. Becky also recorded cows being dragged onto trucks with chains and others left unattended and frozen to the ground.

In the wake of the work we were doing at Lancaster Stockyards, I came to know other activists across the United States who were also concerned about farmed animals. I started to visit other stockyards and shoot video documenting the conditions I found there, just as Becky did. Becky sent me some of her tapes, and together we approached stockyard officials and asked them to do what Lancaster had promised: to refuse downers at their gates. Becky and I held several meetings with the management of the South St. Paul stockyard. They claimed they understood our position and concerns and, in fact, agreed with us. They had a no-downer policy, they told us, on weekends, when the stockyard was not selling animals but did receive them. We wanted one in place full-time.

We went back and forth for a while, with us asking for policy changes and improved enforcement and them responding that it was really someone else's problem. "We can't change this. It's up to somebody else," they told us. "We need to educate the farmers." To Becky and me, that wasn't enough, so we let the stockyard's management know we'd be holding a demonstration at the stockyard on Memorial Day 1991, modeled after the one we'd held in Lancaster three years before.

By this time, Farm Sanctuary was becoming known to both the agricultural community and members of the media, with whom Becky and I shared clips of her video footage. As the day of the demonstration approached, the national and regional media, as well as farm publications, began to cover the issue of downed animals at South St. Paul and other U.S. stockyards. The *NBC Nightly News* with Tom Brokaw and the network's newsmagazine show *Expose* (the forerunner of *Dateline*) both aired stories that reached a national audience. Meanwhile, in its April edition, *The Farmer,* a publication for the midwestern agricultural community, reported that many feared our demonstration would "give the entire livestock industry a black eye." Also around this time, the editor of the Wisconsin-based magazine *Country Today* wrote in a farming journal that the issue of downed animals was a legitimate problem the industry needed to address.

So intense was the pressure that shortly before Memorial Day, the head of the United Stockyards Corporation called a press conference and announced the formal adoption of a no-downer policy at all its stockyards, including South St. Paul. With this decision, the largest stockyards across the United States now had official no-downer policies. It was too late to cancel the demonstration, so we turned it into a celebration. Over a thousand people turned out to hear Farm Sanctuary's new message: "United Stockyards has done this. But there are still downed animals across the country. We're now taking the campaign national. We're going to Washington, D.C." And so we did.

The Path to Washington

Needless to say, our days on the road with the Dead and the Deadheads were a far cry from our political work in Washington, D.C. We found the hallways of the Capitol well worn by the shoes of the agribusiness lobby. The only federal law that limited the suffering of farm animals was the Humane Slaughter Act, enacted in 1958. It required that cattle, pigs, and other mammals, but specifically not birds, be rendered insensible to pain before being shackled and having their throats cut. It was encouraging to know that despite the inadequacies of the law, even half a century ago farm animals had advocates among the American public. "If I went by mail," said President Dwight D. Eisenhower before he signed the act into law, "I'd think no one was interested in anything but humane slaughter."

A generation later, we had a chance to support a much-needed, long-overdue second piece of national legislation to protect farm animals. The downer issue had gained some important supporters. The NBC News story on downer cows had drawn the attention of national legislators, including Senator Daniel Akaka of Hawaii. Senator Akaka agreed that treating incapacitated animals harshly was wrong and decided to introduce a bill to put a national ban on the practice. In 1991, I went to Washington to discuss the downer issue with members of Senator Akaka's staff.

Early in 1992, the House of Representatives' Agriculture Committee's Subcommittee on Livestock, Dairy, and Poultry invited me to testify at hearings it held to address the handling of downed animals at stockyards. I also appeared on CNN's *Larry King Live* with John Lang, then president and CEO of the Livestock Conservation Institute, to discuss the abuse of animals in stockyards and on factory farms. Lang contended that instances of downed animals were few and that Farm Sanctuary had exploited the issue and made it seem a bigger problem than it actually was. At the end of the segment, Lang agreed that I could visit his family's dairy farm and inspect the operations. But when the cameras were off it was a different story, and subsequent phone calls requesting a visit were never returned.

The need for federal legislation became clear when, about a year after United Stockyards announced it would no longer accept downed animals at its seven stockyards, a Farm Sanctuary investigator visited each facility and found downers at three locations. One cow had been left in a dumpster in terrible shape. A local television reporter confronted the president of United Stockyards about the incident and other violations of its own no-downer policy. In each case, he admitted that the animal had not been treated properly and that United Stockyards had a problem. Farm Sanctuary used the results of this investigation to support our case that stockyards' voluntary policies did not work and that laws were necessary, especially when inertia, convenience, or economic interest made it likely the policies would be ignored.

As the Downed Animal Protection Act was being drafted, the U.S. Department of Agriculture (USDA), forced by growing public concern about downers, used a division of the agency, the Packers and Stockyards Administration, to enforce language in the 1921 Packers and Stockyards Act. The act was originally passed to ensure that livestock markets treated their customers fairly and contained a provision to ensure that reasonable care was taken to maintain the quality and value of animals entering stockyards to be sold. While the provision was probably intended to inhibit stockyards from unfairly neglecting individual farmers' animals, the P&SA decided to embrace a different reading. Leaving downed animals to suffer and die, they decided, did not constitute "reasonable care."

The P&SA sent a letter to stockyards across the United States noting that the handling of downed animals had received "considerable, and unfavorable, attention in the media," and suggesting that because stockyards might have difficulty handling downed animals humanely, "the most effective solution is to refuse to accept such livestock." The letter also announced that the P&SA was commencing a surveillance program to review stockyards' handling practices, services, and facilities. Finally, it put stockyards on notice that "evidence of improper handling of livestock at stockyards uncovered by these investigative activities will be dealt with through appropriate corrective action by the Agency."

At last, a government agency was willing to take responsibility for downed animals and make sure others did as well. Soon the P&SA had investigators in the field and began bringing charges against stockyards for violations. One stockyard in Amarillo, Texas, the agency stated, had failed to provide reasonable care to a disabled cow. According to the agency's report, the cow was unloaded at the stockyard "by fastening one end of a chain around the neck of the animal and the other end to a stationary post, and driving the truck from under the animal, causing it to be dragged across the floor of the trailer, up a cleated ramp, and dropped approximately four feet out the back of the trailer to the ground." The cow was alive and conscious, but unable to stand, at the stockyard for two days before it was "destroyed." In another instance, a downed cow at a Tennessee stockyard was, the agency reported, left lying in a muddy outdoor pen in freezing rain without food or water for about two days. In this case, the stockyard agreed to pay a fine of $750.

Over the next few years, I worked with P&SA officials, reporting cases of downed animals Farm Sanctuary came across in the course of our investigations. This arrangement with the P&SA was important because although Senator Akaka and Representative Gary Ackerman of New York had introduced the Downed Animal Protection Act into the Senate and the House in 1992, it had yet to become law. Throughout the 1990s, as we attempted to address various problems associated with the transportation and marketing of downed animals, the bill moved from solely concerning itself with stockyards and auctions to dealing with animals at slaughterhouses as well. There was no law in place, but in spite of that, some large fast-food chains, including McDonald's, Burger King, and Wendy's, stopped using meat from downed cattle, while the Agricultural Marketing Service of the USDA adopted a policy against buying meat from downed cattle for the nation's school lunch program.

Unfortunately, the P&SA's involvement in the downer issue came to an abrupt end. In 1997, the P&SA, now called GIPSA (the Grain Inspection, Packers, and Stockyards Administration), had documentation of a downed cow who'd been left for dead at a stockyard near Phoenix, Arizona, with no shelter, food, or water on a day when the temperature reached a scorching 100 degrees. When GIPSA attempted to sanction the stockyard, the stockyard took the matter to court. An administrative law judge ruled against GIPSA, stating that nothing in the Packers and Stockyards Act indicated it was designed to protect a cow, and the Secretary of Agriculture wasn't given any jurisdiction by the act to "prevent an animal's suffering, injury or death." Because the downed cow had no economic value, the judge's argument went, the law's reasonable-care requirement to maintain the "quality and value" of the animal didn't apply. GIPSA appealed the ruling, but its request was formally denied. GIPSA's surveillance role had come to an end.

This turn of events, dispiriting as it was, gave new energy to our efforts to see the federal Downed Animal Protection Act become law. But while the act had important supporters, including Senator Akaka, Representative Ackerman, and Senator Tom Harkin from the farm state of Iowa, it also had strong opponents. Among them were then Senator Jesse Helms of North Carolina and Representative Charles Stenholm of Texas, who did their best to stifle the act in their respective agriculture committees in both houses of Congress. They succeeded.

The Rise of Mad Cow Disease

By the early 1990s, the issue of downed animals in the food supply reached beyond concerns about animal cruelty—there was danger of contamination of the food supply itself. Evidence from the United Kingdom and the United States suggested the potential risks of disease for people eating the meat of downed animals, including mad cow disease (the popular name for bovine spongiform encephalopathy, or BSE). BSE causes animals to lose control of their motor functions, froth at the mouth, collapse, and eventually die. Autopsies reveal that the cows' brains are punctuated by holes, resembling a sponge (hence *spongiform*). In 1986, Britain identified the first case of mad cow disease; eventually almost two hundred thousand cattle in the United Kingdom would be affected by BSE.

In 1996 the British government announced a probable link between BSE and a form of human dementia: variant Creutzfeldt-Jakob disease (vCJD). Three people in the United Kingdom died of vCJD in 1995. The likely cause was meat from cattle that had been fed the remains of other cattle infected with BSE. The fear of a human epidemic led the British government to ban the feeding of cow remains to other cows in 1996. A year later, the U.S. government issued its own ban, similar to the United Kingdom's but not as extensive.

Even before the first case of vCJD was identified in the United Kingdom, Farm Sanctuary, Michael Greger (a medical doctor and writer, now on staff at the Humane Society of the United States), and others were already concerned about the potential for downed animals to be infected with a variant of BSE. In 1993, despite the U.S. government's assurances that BSE wasn't present in the U.S. cattle population, Dr. Richard Marsh of the Department of Animal Health and Biomedical Sciences at the University of Wisconsin, Madison, published research that suggested the presence of an "unrecognized BSE-like disease in the United States." Marsh and other scientists hypothesized that the deaths of thousands of mink from transmissible mink encephalopathy (TME) on midwestern mink farms was linked to the minks' feed, which was made up largely of downed cows.

A year later, a study published in the *Journal of Infectious Diseases* showed that the disease agent responsible for scrapie, a sheep disease similar to BSE, which has been in the United States for decades, could also infect cattle. Scientists infected calves with scrapie and found that after twelve months they "became severely lethargic and demonstrated clinical signs of motor neuron dysfunction that were manifest as progressive stiffness, posterior paresis, general weakness, and permanent recumbency." In other words, they became downed cows.

Because it was so hard to get the Downed Animal Protection Act passed into law—even in the context of mad cow and vCJD in Britain—Farm Sanctuary petitioned the USDA to prohibit the use of diseased animals for human food. Downed animals were by definition diseased, we argued, and therefore, under existing laws, could not legally be sold for human consumption. Furthermore, since downers were a small percentage of farmed animals being slaughtered, keeping them out of the food supply would cause little economic hardship to the animal agriculture industry. Nobody keeps track or knows the number of downed animals in the United States, but the USDA has estimated there may be around 195,000 downed cattle each year.

Even so, the USDA denied our petition—apparently it was acceptable to allow diseased animals into the human food supply. Indeed, their letter made it clear that the practice was common and well established (and all legal under the governing law, the Federal Meat Inspection Act, and pertinent regulations enforced by the USDA's Food Safety Inspection Service). Responding to our concerns that downed animals with various diseases, including mad cow disease, could, if they entered the food supply, threaten consumers' health, the USDA said that BSE had not been detected in the United States "despite active surveillance efforts for several years." This would have been less discomforting if the USDA *had* been engaged in "active surveillance efforts." In reality, it had been ignoring credible evidence indicating the presence of BSE or variants of the disease in the United States for years.

The agency also said that the risk of BSE or other potential diseases spreading to people through the consumption of red meat was "extremely remote" but, it conceded, possible. The USDA dismissed our economic argument, writing that condemning meat from a carcass with "any degree of disease" would have a serious economic impact. Then, astonishingly, it added that "a large percent of the livers of livestock (greater than ten percent) are condemned because of disease conditions."

We had to find out more, and soon after, we obtained thousands of slaughterhouse records through the Freedom of Information Act. We were astounded to find that animals with abscesses, gangrene, hepatitis, pneumonia, peritonitis, and malignant lymphoma were approved for human food, and all of them were entering the food supply. We thought this would come as news to consumers, too.

In rejecting our petition, the USDA claimed that veterinarians working for the Food Safety Inspection Service knew how to distinguish among different conditions that would cause a cow to go down, using clinical observation, an adequate history, and appropriate laboratory test evaluations. But USDA vets are *not* equipped to perform such observations. As we saw for ourselves, USDA records on downed animals at slaughterhouses appeared to be written hastily and sloppily. Some were illegible or incomplete, while others had serious mistakes and discrepancies. Sometimes the same animal was reported as being both "passed" *and* "condemned" for human food. Inspectors also apparently changed their minds about these designations on the spot. Since downed animals were automatically considered suspect and thus subject to more thorough and careful examinations than other animals, it was particularly disconcerting to find these records so wholly inadequate.

As you can imagine, we were far from satisfied with the USDA's response and its reluctance to take any action. Mad cow disease was a reality in the United Kingdom. Evidence suggested that downed cattle were at a greater risk for BSE. So we felt the only responsible thing to do was to take the USDA to court. Our initial suit was dismissed, but we appealed, and in December 2003 a federal court in New York ruled that our case could go forward. That was the plan, at least.

Understanding the Real Risks
of Downed Animals

Throughout those years of work on national policies and legislation, much of it extremely frustrating since we had little to show for it, I continued visiting stockyards and documenting the treatment of downed animals and was reminded of what we were trying to prevent.

In 2002, ten years after the Downed Animal Protection Act had been introduced in Congress, Senators Akaka and Patrick Leahy of Vermont, and Representatives Ackerman and Amo Houghton of New York, saw to it that a provision on downed animals was added to both the Senate and the House's farm bills. The amendment would prohibit the marketing and dragging of downed animals at stockyards and require incapacitated animals to be humanely euthanized.

Congressman Ackerman summed up Farm Sanctuary's nearly fifteen years of work on the floor of the House of Representatives: "As I stand here before you . . . a frail, day-old calf is dragged through an auction ring by a rope tied to its back leg while another calf, nearly comatose, is left in a corner dying. These are downed animals." He continued: "They make up nearly one-tenth of one percent of the market. And not to euthanize them just because they are of no value when they are dead at marketplace is indeed a sin." He concluded that the amendment would protect both the downed animals themselves and public health, making the amendment "an appropriate remedy to an unnecessary and inexcusable practice."

The House's farm bill passed first, then the Senate's, the latter with a provision almost identical to the downed animal language in the House version. This was a major achievement. Not since the Humane Slaughter Act more than forty years earlier had legislation protecting farm animals passed both houses of Congress.

But our elation was short-lived. After a conference committee met to reconcile differences between the House and Senate versions of the bill, powerful legislators hostile to the downed animal provision pulled it from the bill. In its place, the conference report that emerged from the committee called for the secretary of agriculture to "investigate and submit to Congress a report" on the downed animal issue. We had been at it for fifteen years! How much more information and documentation, we wondered, could Congress possibly need? The conference report was then sent back to the full House and Senate for final approval. Farm Sanctuary and other animal protection groups fought its passage, concerned about the gutting of the downed animal legislation, but despite these efforts, both the Senate and the House approved the farm bill conference report.

It was clear that we needed a stronger voice in Congress, to make sure our constituents were heard. Since then, Humane USA, a political action committee for the humane movement, has been established, and animal advocates are more sophisticated about how things work in Washington. For instance, one effective way of getting something through Congress is to attach language to appropriations bills—the bills governing how federal funds are spent.

To his great credit, Representative Ackerman refused to give up on downed animals. In 2003, he, along with Representative Steven LaTourette of Ohio, proposed an amendment to the 2004 Agriculture Appropriations bill that would prohibit the USDA from spending money to oversee the slaughter of downed animals for human food. By cutting off the funds (a fairly common Washington legislative tactic), the practice could, we hoped, be ended. A similar amendment was introduced in the Senate. If approved, the amendments could possibly prevent downers from being slaughtered and entering the human food supply, or at least prevent U.S. taxpayers from paying for this to happen.

Once again, we came very close. But, while the Senate passed the measure, the House defeated it by a vote of 202 to 199, in large measure due to the efforts of Representative Stenholm. Our effort to enact sensible reform had been thwarted, and it was a huge disappointment.

Soon, however, evidence of a danger to consumers overpowered legislative maneuvering. On December 24, 2003, the USDA announced the first case of mad cow disease in the United States, reportedly found in a downed cow in Washington State. The USDA then proceeded to launch a media blitz to assure consumers in the United States and around the world that U.S. beef was safe to eat. Naturally, Farm Sanctuary and other groups redoubled our campaign to remove downed animals from the food supply. Those in Congress who had fought these efforts were eerily silent during the public debate. Six days later, on December 30, the USDA implemented an interim policy against downed cattle entering the human food supply, which was made permanent in 2007. Less than two weeks before the mad cow case was confirmed, Farm Sanctuary had won a court decision that reinstated our lawsuit against the USDA, but with the new policy in place, the case was soon settled. The USDA explicitly acknowledged that downed cows are more likely to have a range of diseases than healthy cattle, including mad cow.

While we were pleased the USDA finally reversed its longstanding position that consuming meat from downed cows poses no threat to human health, it was, unfortunately, a reactive measure, taken only after mad cow was identified. Alarmingly, a 2006 report from the Office of the Inspector General found that downed cows were still being slaughtered and used for human food in violation of the USDA's no-downer policy. We'd like to see the ban strengthened and better enforced, and we are also encouraging the USDA to broaden it to apply not only to downed cows but to pigs (downed pigs are a growing problem), sheep, and all other sick livestock. But the industry is still reluctant to do the right thing. Despite several additional cases of mad cow found in North American cattle since 2003, the livestock industry continues seeking to weaken the ban on the use of downed cattle for human food.

The USDA and agribusiness have strong economic incentives to turn a blind eye to mad cow disease—and, for that matter, other diseases in farmed animals. One is the huge export market for U.S. beef, which was rattled when BSE was confirmed. Agriculture adopted a "don't look, don't find" approach, choosing to ignore and perhaps even hide evidence that a variant of mad cow disease had been in the United States since at least the early 1990s. Once again, producers seem to be putting their interests above the health of the public, the well-being of their animals, and the long-term viability of their industry. Sad to say, short-term financial gains still blind agribusiness and government regulators to long-term consequences.

Whatever the reason for not testing all or a majority of cattle, the

United States is falling behind in tracking cattle who may have BSE, according to a *Wall Street Journal* article from June 2006. There is, says the paper, still "no national ID system for most farm animals, including chickens and beef cattle." In July 2006, the USDA announced it was slashing funding for its program to test for mad cow disease by almost *90 percent.* Under the new policy, only about forty thousand animals a year will be tested, a tiny fraction of the nearly thirty-five million cattle slaughtered annually.

At the same time, the U.S. government is discouraging producers who want to do more rigorous tests. When the Kansas-based beef processor Creekstone Farms proposed testing all its beef cattle for BSE, the USDA refused it permission to do so. The government agency claimed that universal testing would not increase food safety, since, it argued, BSE is not easily detected in younger cattle. While it's possible the government thinks it's protecting the U.S. food supply, I believe the USDA is concerned that if every animal was tested they'd find more cases of mad cow disease and its true prevalence would become more well known.

There is some good news. At least for now, there's no longer a financial incentive to keep downed cows alive and drag them onto and off trucks to be slaughtered, because they aren't currently allowed to be sold for human consumption. But there's also bad news. Renderers are receiving federal funds to test downed cows' brains for potential BSE. Some renderers don't like the smell of dead carcasses; they want the animals transported alive. In some cases, this means that live downed cows are being left to suffer for hours or days before they are killed. Twenty years after Farm Sanctuary began working on the downer issue, sick animals are still being left to suffer on farms, in stockyards, and in slaughterhouses, and, apart from cows (theoretically), are still making their way into the food supply. Although we have made progress on some aspects of the downed animal problem, the underlying perception of these animals as commodities rather than as individuals with feelings and the capacity to suffer hasn't changed. That is a longer and greater struggle.

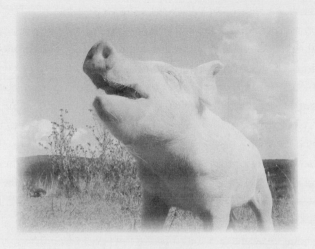

Rudy

PROFILE: TRUFFLES, RUDY, AND TERRIN

Truffles was a very young piglet, weighing no more than twenty pounds, when she was loaded onto a hot, crowded truck to be shipped off to a "finishing" farm where she would be fattened for slaughter. Luckily for her, she fell out of the truck into heavy traffic on I-69 in Indiana. A woman driving in the opposite direction saw the pig fall and knew she had to stop and save her. She pulled over, ran across the median, scooped the terrified piglet into her arms, and safely placed a bruised and bloody Truffles in the backseat of her car. The woman then contacted a Farm Sanctuary member, who agreed to foster the piglet until she could be transported to Watkins Glen, where she lives today.

Rudy was also picked up in Indiana after a truck driver spotted him wandering around a parking lot off I-74 shortly after a truck full of piglets pulled out. Rudy was taken to the local animal shelter, where his only company was dogs in the adjacent cages, which only made him more scared and distressed. Animal control officers planned to give him to a nearby farmer to raise him for food. Luckily, hearing from a TV news report what was going to happen to Rudy, Farm Sanctuary members intervened, and when the farmer missed the deadline to pick up Rudy, the piglet made his way to the same foster home as Truffles.

By the time Rudy and Truffles arrived at Watkins Glen, they were inseparable. Rudy was and still is very shy. When he first came, he was terrified of the caregivers, who were initially unable to get anywhere near him. It took a long while for him to trust us and for us to get to know him. Rudy and Truffles then teamed up with Terrin, another pig found on the side of an Ohio highway (she had apparently fallen off an overcrowded trailer), to form a mini-herd. The three of them love hanging out together. We give them a special diet that will make them less prone to weight gain, and they are still very agile, unlike some of our older pigs who are so big they have trouble moving around.

Truffles is inquisitive, friendly, and the boldest of the three. She loves to greet visitors with a happy grunt. She's also very confident and will sniff you over to take your measure. She particularly loves making mud holes with her snout. Terrin is sweet, very kind, and intensely protective of Truffles and Rudy, especially when we're giving them veterinary care. Rudy is high-strung, so we are careful to avoid situations that make him anxious. If you come to the farm and he decides he wants to undo your shoelaces, as has happened with some of our visitors, then you should probably let him. Truffles also loves to untie shoelaces and is very good at it. All three pigs love to play in and turn over the soil, enjoying the smell and touch and taste of the earth as they search for roots and bugs. We give them inflatable balls to play with, some with handles, which they use to whack each other.

There's one thing that Rudy, Truffles, and Terrin have in common with nearly all the other pigs: they can't stand the sound of clanking metal. Even though they were very young, they must remember what it was like to be crowded behind metal slats on that transport truck. They hate the very sound of trucks. When the UPS truck drives up to the farm, they run and hide. It's a reminder of how sensitive and intelligent pigs are and that, while they may forgive, they don't forget.

CHAPTER FOUR

Watkins Glen

"You guys got college degrees and you're out there doing *what?*" In my mind, I could see my parents rolling their eyes as I talked with them on the phone. They thought Lorri and I were nuts, and who could blame them? By the late 1980s, only a few years after Farm Sanctuary had been founded, we were living in a retired school bus in the middle of Pennsylvania with no toilet, no mechanized equipment, and a growing family of farm animals we had rescued from stockyards, among them Maya; Hope, an injured pig we'd rescued from Lancaster Stockyards; Hilda; and Jellybean, another rescued sheep who became Hilda's good friend. Throughout her life, Hilda remained shy around people and could always be found near Jellybean. I often watched Hilda and Jellybean graze and wander through the pasture and felt happy to provide them with a safe haven.

We thought it was important that, as individual beings, the animals have unique names. At Farm Sanctuary, the animals would be a "who" and not a "that," a "he" or "she" and not an "it." To this day, every animal who comes to live at Farm Sanctuary or whom we place in another home is given a name. Sometimes they're named after people, as Hilda is. Sometimes the names, such as Hope, reflect the spirit they embody. Sometimes, as in the case of Maya, the name just seems to fit. Once, we took in a number of calves rescued from veal production and named them all after famous vegetarians, including Albert, as in Schweitzer, and Leo, as in Tolstoy. Billy Martin was a goat with a certain attitude, so we named him after that notoriously cantankerous Yankees' baseball team manager. Sometimes we'd name the animals for the places we found them; other names came from an earthier source. Sheep droppings resemble jelly-beans, and that's how Jellybean got her name.

Unlike our legislative efforts, rescuing animals provided tangible sol-ace. We were doing something concrete that was making a difference for these individuals. As the number of sheep, calves, pigs, and chickens in our care grew, the shortcomings of the row house on Stroud Street in Wilmington became all too clear. We needed more space if Farm Sanctu-ary was going to continue to be a real place of sanctuary.

Sometimes a coincidence or casual conversation can change the course of your life, and our next move was the result of tofu. Back then I was a pretty good cook, and to supplement our income from the veggie dog sales at Grateful Dead concerts, we also catered parties and events in the Brandywine region of Pennsylvania. Since this was vegetarian ca-tering—and predated the explosion of vegetarian gourmet cooking—I used a lot of tofu. For one fancy brunch, I remember making scrambled tofu and Thanksgiving-style stuffing (a great combination, if you're won-dering). Through our catering work, we got to know Warren Reynolds, whose family owned a dairy farm. When Warren inherited it, he turned the dairy operation into a soy milk production facility that also dabbled in making tofu. When I went to buy tofu at Warren's farm, he and I got to talking. He was a warmhearted guy and sympathetic to our efforts. During one of our conversations, Warren offered us the use of about three acres of his farm in Avondale, Pennsylvania, as a sanctuary and a home.

We leapt at the chance. Warren's farm was a thirty-minute drive from Wilmington and about an hour from Lancaster. We could easily travel between the farm, the Farm Sanctuary office, which we kept at Stroud Street, and the stockyards, and still have time to take care of the ever-increasing number of animals.

The "tofu farm," as I called it, was a real do-it-yourself enterprise. In the donated school bus we called home, a bucket served as the toilet. After a year or so, one of our supporters sponsored a Porta Potti, which, when it was installed, seemed luxurious indeed. We used an old milking parlor as an education center and converted a former dairy barn into a multi-animal barn. We took out the curved metal dividers that had served as stalls, and created three sections where different animals could be kept at night and when it was cold. We also fenced in a little area outside the barn as pasture.

Although I look back now with some affection for the simplicity of that life, all of what we did was out of necessity, not some high-minded adventure. In fact, that school bus got pretty cramped. In those early days, I cut plywood with a hand saw because we didn't have an electric saw and dug four-foot-deep ditches with a pick and shovel. I installed a water system and electricity and built a set of small houses for the animals to use as shelters when they were outside. Although I wasn't a kid from the country, I did have some relevant experience. In addition to having a farming gene, I may have had a handyman gene, too: my father's father was a carpenter who moved to Hollywood to work on movie sets in the 1930s. Growing up, I'd had a wooden tree house, and I'd helped my father convert some of our garage space into a much-needed bedroom. As children, my siblings and I all helped out in the family business. Like kids who grow up on a farm, we learned, almost without trying, how things were done.

Despite their astonishment, my parents weren't openly critical of what I was doing. They tried to be supportive, but I knew they weren't terribly impressed by my choices. But for me it all felt right, and rewarding in the best way. Ours was a simple, visceral reaction to callous cruelty, and I could see how I was making a difference. Animals such as Hilda, Hope, and Raquel, another pig who'd been discarded at Lancaster Stockyards, were now enjoying life. Just think what it means when helpless creatures spend their entire existence in the dark, tortured world of the factory farm, denied nourishing food, the companionship of one another, straw to lie on, and the warmth of the sun. For them, that confinement, fear, and privation are the whole world, all they will ever know of life.

Of course, the scale of the problem was huge, and it's only gotten bigger. Then, as now, we couldn't rescue every farmed animal in need. Temple Grandin, the noted expert on animal behavior, has said that in industrialized animal agriculture "bad has become normal." I couldn't agree more. I was outraged at the system I saw firsthand. "How on earth could this happen?" I asked myself over and over again. "How can animals be so profoundly disrespected? How can injured and sick animals be treated literally as garbage? How can people accept this as the way business is done?"

I felt deeply for the animals, but I was also concerned for the people who had created and lived in this cruel, irrational system that was undermining farming's integrity. As we documented conditions, some of our volunteers and I had intense confrontations with farm people at stockyards in Pennsylvania, Minnesota, and other places. I never enjoyed these. Nor did I enjoy recording the practices I witnessed. Rescuing downed animals from the stockyards and seeing them recuperate was grounding and healing. It helped me deal with my sadness and frustration. It also helped keep me looking forward. Each action led to another task that had to be done.

A Permanent Home

All too soon, the space at the tofu farm proved inadequate for our needs. We were bursting at the seams, and while Warren had been incredibly generous, we realized we needed a more permanent place for the animals, a place Farm Sanctuary owned and could remain in for years to come.

Our experiences on Stroud Street in Wilmington had shown us the potential for a farm animal sanctuary that people could actually visit. Neighborhood kids would stick their heads over the fence of the row house and ask about Hilda and Jellybean and the others, including our first flock of hens. Farm animals were exotic creatures to these children. The kids came by often, excited by whom they might find in our backyard. "What animals have you got this week?" they'd ask. We began to think of the educational potential for Farm Sanctuary. If we stimulated people's curiosity and made it possible for them to meet sheep, cows, pigs, and chickens, their empathy for farmed animals might naturally grow.

I began scanning the real estate section of agricultural publications looking for a new home. Not surprisingly, given the difficulties family farms have competing against the agribusiness giants, I saw a lot of ads. A supporter offered us land near Watertown, New York, for free, but it was forested, and we didn't want to cut down a forest to create a farm.

One day I saw a property for sale in Watkins Glen, New York, in the hills of Schuyler County, about a five-hour drive northwest of New York

City. The ad listed the property as 175 acres, a seven-bedroom house, and barns, and said it came with tractors and other equipment. Compared with the other farms for sale, it had the most acreage for the lowest price and included a big old farmhouse. We could move in and start working right away. Or so we thought.

"You know, it's hard to sell this place," the real estate agent said when we visited. I could see why. Although the house, which had been built in stages beginning in the mid-1800s, had white pillars in front, as well as a certain elegance, an enormous pile of garbage in the front yard greeted us as we drove up. Later we acquired a photo of the family who'd built it; a man leans against one of the pillars, smoking a cigar, as if to say, "I've arrived." It was clear on our first visit that the farm had fallen on hard times since, and we soon found out why. The current owner had retired from a career in the railroad industry and wanted to be a farmer. He set up a pig operation along with some crops. He pushed the animals and the land hard but didn't do very well. One day he was out on his tractor plowing a field when the plow stuck. He didn't stop the tractor in time and it flipped over on top of him, trapping his leg against the plow. The farmer lost that leg, fell into a depression, and eventually killed himself. The family's fortunes went downhill from there. By the time we were looking to buy the farm, one son was on his way to jail and a teenage daughter had just become a single mom. It was all very unfortunate.

The house reflected the story. The glass in the front door was missing. Honey dripped from a jar left on its side in the kitchen, and we had to chisel grease off the stove. In the basement I found an old freezer that hadn't worked for a long time. When I opened it up, I practically passed out: inside was a dead deer that no doubt had been there for months. The barns were disintegrating, and the tractors and the equipment didn't work. And we'd thought the school bus in Avondale was rough! Nevertheless, the farm had substantial acreage, an old hay barn, and three other outbuildings, plus the house, and was the best farm for the price that we saw. The owner was asking $110,000. We got it for $100,000.

Our growing community of supporters helped make the purchase possible. In the mid- to late 1980s, the animal rights movement in the United States was beginning. People for the Ethical Treatment of

Animals (PETA) was hitting its stride. Many activities were under way: demonstrations, investigations, and public education. When we could, we attended national animal rights conferences in Washington, D.C., where we spoke with many of the movement's current and emerging leaders about what we were doing. (I remember meeting Wayne Pacelle, now president and CEO of the Humane Society of the United States, at one of these conferences when he was still a student at Yale.) For the first time, there seemed to be a critical mass of animal activists. While there was activism against the fur trade, hunting, and vivisection (experimentation on animals), little attention was being focused on the issue of factory farming. When we described what we were doing, we found a number of allies—individual activists as well as groups—who were more than willing to help support Farm Sanctuary's work.

Soon after we started Farm Sanctuary, some of the most dedicated of these supporters organized fund-raising walkathons for farm animals. In October 1989, a series of these walkathons in New York, Philadelphia, and elsewhere raised $25,000 to help us put a down payment on the farm. My mom and dad—graciously putting their doubts aside—secured a loan for the remaining $75,000, which we later paid off. We were thrilled—and had our work cut out for us given the state of the farm. As we and a small group of volunteers laid out fences and pipes, built new structures, and renovated the existing ones, we liked to think we were changing the character and karma of the property.

By the summer of 1990 we were ready to bring the animals up from Pennsylvania to their new home. They were about 150 strong, including quite a few hens rescued from battery cages where they'd been confined with barely enough room to move. At the Watkins Glen farm all the animals had substantially more living space in both the barns and the pastures than they'd ever had before. They were soon rooting in the dirt, exploring the fields and the trees, or just lolling around, enjoying the warm summer days.

For the human residents of Farm Sanctuary, things were a little rougher. Blanche Kent, an animal caregiver we met in Pennsylvania, several interns, and Lorri and I lived together in the farmhouse, where we also had the office. We used one room as a basic bed-and-breakfast. We all shared the kitchen, the bathroom, and the office. Our bedroom was smaller than the average undergraduate's dorm room, smaller even than our "bedroom" on the old school bus on the tofu farm. It was also under the eaves, which meant I couldn't stand upright except near the door.

The first new barn we built was for the cows. We ran water and electric lines to it, which also made it a logical place for another kind of living space—a loft apartment for me and Lorri. We moved in about a year after we bought the property. The human habitat in the loft was enclosed and insulated, with a little porch open to the barn. In the evenings, we'd sit on that porch munching on tortilla chips. The cows—about twenty of them by this time—didn't seem to mind. It was almost like a whale watch. From our perch, we'd look down on the cows' broad backs. Sometimes they would look up at us and eat the chips from our outstretched hands. One of the things I've learned from the farmed animals we've rescued and cared for over the years is that if they're treated cruelly or harshly, they'll grow fearful and may act out. We were a friendly human presence, and the cows knew the difference. The barn was their place and the loft was our place, and we were both at home.

I loved living in the cow barn. In general, cows tend to be easygoing, but they're big animals, and when a few of them rubbed up against the barn posts, the whole loft shook. At night we'd hear them rustling and breathing as they ruminated, chewing their cud. On clear evenings, they were quiet. But on stormy nights, the cows would come stampeding into the barn. They weren't so much afraid as fired up, as if they'd been electrified by the energy. You could really feel it.

Cattle move with the earth's rhythms in a way that's hard to describe. At times, I've even heard them breathe sympathetically with people who are in a state of heightened emotion. Like us, they enjoy pleasant weather, and I've seen cattle in a state of bliss as they graze on sweet clover or grasses at certain times of the year. After a long winter in Watkins Glen, when they've spent the better part of the last few months inside the barns eating hay, the cattle relish the spring days. They kick up their feet, run, and jump. At the peak of the summer heat they hang out under the trees enjoying the shade. I often wonder what the world would be like if we did more of this ourselves. "Every person and every living creature," Leo Tolstoy wrote, "has a sacred right to the gladness of springtime."

Mending Fences, Changing Minds

When we first arrived in Watkins Glen, I think most of the farmers in the area saw us as a threat. Farm Sanctuary was a foreign idea to many people, including our neighbors whose business was animal agriculture. Someone apparently warned them that we had designs on their animals—that our intention was nothing short of stealing them away. The farming economy at that time in upstate New York, as well as the region's overall economy, was depressed, while we were constructing new barns. We were rescuing animals and letting them live. And we were growing as an organization. By contrast, like many independent American farmers, the farmers in and around Watkins Glen were eking out a living raising animals to be slaughtered in barns that were falling down. The irony wasn't lost on them or on us.

Part of the tension between us stemmed from a clash of cultures and worldviews—not unlike our dealings with agribusiness veterinarians, who often told us that the cost of providing medical treatment far outweighed an animal's market value, and recommended against it. We explained (again and again) that we valued the animal as an individual, not a commodity. (A discussion about the status of animals as something other than property is now under way among many veterinarians and veterinarians' associations.) They'd look at me skeptically, but most would eventually provide the needed care. More than once, visiting vets have been so impressed by the good health of the Farm Sanctuary animals that they suggested we should go into the business of raising calves. I had a chuckle at that.

The farmers in our corner of upstate New York also couldn't understand why we'd spend so much money on animals we weren't going to sell as food. And yet they recognized a well-run operation, even if the traditional output was zero. "I've never seen such a clean farm," one farmer commented. "I've never seen such healthy animals," opined another.

At the same time, I appreciated and benefited from the camaraderie that exists among farmers, though I was definitely unconventional. Because I didn't have the lifelong experience my neighbors had from working on their family farms, I was always open to their advice, and over the years I've found many farmers happy to give it. I've learned a lot from them. When we first moved to Watkins Glen, for instance, one of the men who used to live on the land walked the property with me and told me its history. He knew it well and pointed out a natural spring that produced water all year long, a good thing to know. I've revisited that spot many times and drunk fresh water directly from the earth.

The man was very friendly, but although we had some things in common, no one would ever call us kindred spirits. When we reached a tree up on the ridge of the hill, he stopped. "I've hunted from that tree since I was a boy," he said, "and I'd like to keep hunting there."

"Well, you know, we have a different view of things, and we're not going to allow any hunting," I replied. He wasn't happy, but all the same, I've called that tree the "peace tree" ever since.

Since the tractors we had bought with the farm turned out to be nothing more than scrap, we had to find new equipment. Some of what we purchased was brand-new, and some was secondhand from farm auctions. Many farmers in the region—particularly dairy operators—were going out of business and liquidating all of their assets, so there was a lot of equipment for sale and prices were low. At farm auctions, tractors, tools, and implements are displayed and the auctioneer leads buyers from one item to the next, selling them off as he goes along. I could see how stretched the farming community was and could feel the owners' pain. They were giving up a way of life—and for who knew what? Most farmers were desperate for a sale. Human nature being what it is, some people at the auctions regretted the farmer's misfortune, while others were giddy at the bargain prices.

For the most part, the suspicion that greeted us when we first arrived in Watkins Glen is behind us. Over the years, we've shown ourselves to be more than good neighbors. We're a force for good in the community, and there's much more mixing of cultures now. For instance, a relative of one of the farm's former owners works in the Farm Sanctuary office. We have also created a number of jobs for people who used to work on local farms. Some are members of the cleaning crew, while others work in the fields, in construction, as feed suppliers, and as caretakers and administrators. We have even had visitors from the farming world who have come to the Sanctuary, spent some time working with the animals, and left aspiring vegans. I love it when that happens. The place can have that effect on people, and it doesn't come from ponderous lectures. All they have to do is connect with the animals and feel the peaceful spirit in the air.

Some farmers even come to *me* for advice. They ask us to help, for instance, with sick animals they can't take care of. On occasion, we've taken these animals in. Veterinarians have also spread word of our work to farmers, so they know that animals who need help may be able to get it from us. We're mindful, however, of what happened at the Lancaster Stockyards—we don't want to expend resources that enable farmers who fail to treat their animals well. We also don't want to help them raise animals for slaughter. Our policy is that if an animal comes to Farm Sanctuary, that animal begins a new life and is spared forever from exploitation and slaughter.

Since 1990, Farm Sanctuary has invested well over a million dollars in the community around Watkins Glen. We've done an enormous amount of building, which has provided work and income for local businesses. We've put new siding and roofs on some of the barns. We've laid gravel and hired painters, plumbers, electricians, mechanics, well drillers, and water experts. In the early 1990s, we began to build the human part of our organization. We hired staff for the shelter and the office and purchased a house across the street for interns, so more young women and men could come to help out with animal care and farm and office work.

We need plenty of special feed for the animals—high in fiber, chemical-free, and vegan—and we work with a local feed mill to produce and mix it. Naturally, we also employ the services of veterinarians, including several from Cornell University in nearby Ithaca. Ithaca is home to the pioneering Moosewood vegetarian restaurant, a dining destination familiar to many of our visitors. Cornell's College of Agriculture and Life Sciences is one of the leading animal agriculture institutions of its kind in the world, and not long after relocating to Watkins Glen, I enrolled there and obtained a master's degree in agricultural economics.

As soon as we relocated to upstate New York, we launched a visitor and education program that gave people time with the animals and also exposed them to the realities of factory farming. In doing so, we've substantially increased the local tourist economy. Each year, thousands of visitors to Farm Sanctuary also visit the village of Watkins Glen (population approximately two thousand) to take a boat ride on Seneca Lake, eat at restaurants, shop, tour one of the area's many wineries or gorges, or even attend a NASCAR rally. If our B and B cabins are booked, which is most of the time, we refer people to other accommodations in the area. Many of the visitors who come to Farm Sanctuary ask for vegan meals, so a number of Watkins Glen restaurants have added vegan options. The local Chinese restaurant, House of Hong, even has a vegetarian menu. Good Groceries, our community health food store, sells a tasty vegan "happy hen" sandwich, and other food retailers offer vegan cinnamon buns, "ribs," and hoagies named after some of Farm Sanctuary's animal residents.

In March 1993, Burger King launched its BK veggie burger in Watkins Glen after we and some of our visitors urged them to offer a vegan sandwich. Dennis Kessler, the owner of the franchise, was receptive to the idea that there was an economic opportunity he was missing out on. The veggie burger is now a standard menu option at Burger King restaurants across the United States and internationally.

We also changed the local economy in other ways. When we first moved to the farm, our neighbor across the street was, of all things, a fur farmer. He raised foxes in tiny cages. Understandably, our staff and volunteers were upset by his practices, and from time to time they had contentious exchanges. I didn't like what he was doing, either, but I've always found reasoned dialogue more productive than shouting or name-calling. So I treated him with respect, the way I like (and everyone likes) to be treated.

One year, I invited our fur-farming neighbor and his family to one of the summer "hoedowns" we hold annually on the farm for our supporters and the community. The hoedowns feature farm tours, time with the animals (the pigs love their belly rubs), guest speakers, good food, and a Saturday night barn dance. The fox farmer and his wife and sons accepted. During the day he talked with many of our staff and guests, and in the evening his guitar-playing sons joined in with the other musicians around the campfire. Everyone sang together. It was a small thing, but this farmer was being shown some kindness instead of being lambasted for what he was doing to the foxes.

I think that night our neighbor recognized that we had some things in common. Sometime after the hoedown, he stopped by to talk to me. "You know what?" he said. I don't like killing the animals this way." Then he asked, "What kind of vegetables do you like?" He was ready to make a change. We'd given him the opportunity, and an opening, when our staff put their hostilities and judgments on hold. It *is* possible to "love the sinner, hate the sin." Some of the staff later dubbed that hoedown "the peacefest."

The fur farmer stopped breeding foxes so the population wouldn't grow, and then he decided to get out of the business altogether. My guess is that his enterprise wasn't flourishing, so he could have been simply cutting his losses. Whatever the case, at least the cycle of exploitation had ended. I don't think any of us could have predicted what happened next. He opened up a veggies and crafts stand, right across the street from the entrance to Farm Sanctuary. All of which goes to show that violence toward and exploitation of animals are not the only ways to create jobs and wealth. A healthy economy can emerge from peaceful pursuits as well.

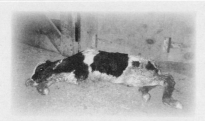

Opie at the stockyards

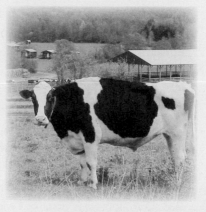

Opie at Farm Sanctuary

PROFILE: OPIE

In 1990, when I was documenting conditions at a stockyard in Bath, New York, I saw a downed calf. By this time I'd seen a large number of downed animals, but it is always deeply disturbing to come across a living being treated with such disregard. This calf had been abandoned in an alleyway, crumpled in a little heap and still wet with afterbirth. He'd probably been born in a dairy facility that morning. More than likely, a truck was scheduled to take other animals from the dairy to the stockyard and the farmer had thrown the calf onto the truck. This stockyard sold calves one day each week, so if the farmer didn't get the calf on the truck that day, he'd have had to wait another seven days to sell him, and there was no financial incentive to wait. A male calf on a dairy farm has no economic value and is often more trouble than he's worth.

It was late fall and freezing cold, and I could see that the calf was in bad shape. To get a sense of how dehydrated calves are, you pinch their skin. If they're adequately hydrated, the skin snaps right back; if not, it goes back very slowly as if it's clay or Play-Doh. The calf's skin wasn't elastic at all. His eyes were sunken and he wasn't responsive. He seemed on the verge of death. I asked a stockyard worker what would happen to the calf, and he said, "I have to bury him later."

I grabbed the calf, put him in the van, and drove to a nearby veterinarian. I walked into the vet's office holding him in my arms. "Can you treat him?" I asked. The vet had worked with local farmers and was not sympathetic to Farm Sanctuary. She glanced at the calf. "He's got less than a five percent chance of survival," she said. "What are you wasting your time for? It makes no economic sense." I looked her straight in the eye. "To us this isn't about economics. It's about an animal who needs help and we want to help him." We went back and forth like this for a while before I finally asked her whether she was going to give him fluids or whether I should go somewhere else. The dehydrated calf was hypothermic—his temperature was almost ten degrees below normal, so low it wouldn't even read on the vet's thermometer. The vet relented and gave the calf fluids intravenously.

I took the calf, whom I later named Opie, back to the farm in Watkins Glen. As with other calves we'd rescued, Opie needed colostrum, which is a mother's first nutrient-rich and immunity-boosting milk. When I approached local dairy farms asking for colostrum they generally gave it to me, assuming that I too was a farmer, which, in a way, I was. A very different kind, perhaps, but whatever the case, we were both raising calves. It's important for calves to develop a suckling reflex so they can start to take milk; if they don't, it's a sign they've lost the will to live. I petted and comforted Opie and put my thumb or finger in his mouth to see if the suckle reflex had started. Thankfully, it had, and he began drinking milk from a bottle. For the next several weeks I spent a good deal of time with him as he recovered.

Since Opie was also on an intravenous drip, we had to make sure the needle stayed in place and the tube didn't get tangled. All this took time and care. Soon, he began to recover physically, but he wasn't thriving. Like any social being, humans included, he needed company of his own kind, as well as physical care. Fragile as he was, I took him out to the cow barn. When he saw the other cattle, he perked up. From that tiny, dehydrated Holstein calf, Opie grew into a huge steer, as a neutered male is known. He now weighs over two thousand pounds. He's tall and has big bones, with huge hips and feet. He's about fifteen years old and well loved by both staff and visitors for his easygoing personality.

People often comment on Opie's size and the size of some of the other steers at Farm Sanctuary whose mothers were dairy cows. A few of them weigh up to three thousand pounds. One reason the steers are so large is that the dairy industry has genetically bred cows for more and more milk production, which has had the unintended result of producing bigger animals. Even though he's a male, Opie has the genetics of a mass production dairy cow. In his prime, Opie, too, weighed about three thousand pounds. As he has gotten older, Opie's legs and joints have started having trouble carrying his weight.

His size has had other consequences. Opie was always an integral member of the cattle herd in Watkins Glen. But once the trouble with his legs began, he had difficulty trying to keep up with the others. Opie now lives with what we call the special needs herd for older or disabled cows, or those who are new to Farm Sanctuary and haven't quite acclimated. But he's happy there. He spends much of his time lying in the pasture, resting his legs, and grazing with Maya, another former downed calf who looked after Opie when he was very young. They'll be together until one of them dies. We've lost a number of steers around Opie's age for the same reason: they're so big, they just can't get up anymore. This is the heartbreaking result of the modern farm industry's obsession with growing animals bigger and genetically programmed to produce more and more.

Opie's joint disease—like human joint disease—is degenerative. Because of his size, there's no fixing his bones. Still, we do everything we can. He gets glucosamine supplements, pain medication when he needs it, and joint injections when his legs get really bad. If the situation gets much worse, we'll have to take a hard look at Opie's quality of life and decide if or when to euthanize him. These are tough issues that all shelters wrestle with. Opie, though, has lived much longer and better than anybody dreamed in that cold stockyard all those years ago.

CHAPTER FIVE

California,
Here We Come

I'm a Californian by birth, and in the early 1990s, something was drawing me west again. As Farm Sanctuary grew more stable financially and the shelter began running pretty smoothly, I started to think more about advocacy on a larger scale. How could we have a national impact on the lives of farmed animals? Part of the answer, I thought, was in California.

Not only is the population of California the largest in the United States, but the state is also number one in terms of agricultural production, the annual value of which exceeds $30 billion. The Golden State usually brings to mind Hollywood, beaches, the "Victorian ladies" of San Francisco, or Silicon Valley. But California was also the setting for much of John Steinbeck's *The Grapes of Wrath;* driven from their farm in Oklahoma by debt and the Dust Bowl, the Joad family headed to California looking for farm work. California is also where Cesar Chavez organized and advocated for exploited farmworkers (Chavez also was a vegan and lent his voice to animal protection efforts). Indeed, many of California's residents still make their living on the land, including a large migrant workforce. Away from California's densely populated urban areas lies some of the country's most productive farmland. Grapes, almonds, strawberries, walnuts, tomatoes, broccoli, peppers, all kinds of greens, and even rice are grown along the coast or in vast fields in the valley that stretches between Bakersfield to the south and Sacramento to the north. While much of the state is desert, extensive irrigation, including water piped in from the Colorado River, makes it possible to grow crops year-round. Given its leading role in American agriculture, California is central to the rapidly expanding market for organic produce.

California is also the nation's top producer of dairy products, having surpassed Wisconsin in milk production in 1993, the year Farm Sanctuary set up shop in California. The state is home to a number of mega-dairies with populations of up to ten thousand cows each—some of the largest dairy facilities in the world. It's the birthplace of the "dry lot" dairy system, which doesn't use pasture. But California's dominance in agriculture may not be sustainable over the long term. As the state's population swells, particularly in cities, the water and land "wars" of the last century are likely to intensify, and the agriculture industry may cash out and move to less populated areas. Already, developers are buying up dairy farms throughout Southern California to build new housing.

Establishing a shelter for rescued farmed animals in California made sense. From there we could help educate more of the American public about industrial agricultural practices, encourage reforms in production and consumer habits, and have a base from which to conduct investigations and rescue and rehabilitate animals throughout the western United States. One of our supporters, a professor at California State University, found available land suitable for a sanctuary near Orland, in the northwest part of California's Central Valley, and donated about a hundred acres to us. We were able to purchase an additional two hundred acres from a local rancher, bringing our total acreage to three hundred.

Farm Sanctuary West

Orland is a small city, with a population of about five thousand located on Interstate 5, the primary north-south thoroughfare on the West Coast, running from Canada to Mexico. And you can't drive more than a few miles without catching sight of a truck hauling livestock, poultry, or other agricultural products. This is an agricultural region, and in and around Orland farmers produce olives, walnuts, almonds, plums, peaches, and rice. There are also many beef and dairy farms nearby, and the road in front of our sanctuary has even been used to herd cattle from pasture to pasture. Our property is in the eastern foothills of the coastal mountain range. From some parts of the farm, if you look to the north on clear days, you can see the snow-capped peak of Mount Shasta, an extinct volcano that rises to more than fourteen thousand feet.

The Orland shelter is about a hundred acres larger than the farm in Watkins Glen. The land is much drier, the landscape is more expansive (with far fewer trees), and for much of the year nature's palette is muted. Although Orland is arid, there is water in the vicinity. We're across the road from the Black Butte Lake Recreation Area. The lake was formed in the 1960s when the Black Butte Dam was completed to manage and store rain and river water for use by nearby communities during the dry months. You can swim and boat in Black Butte Lake, as well as hike and camp in the area. When it gets hot (and it does, with temperatures in the summer often reaching the high nineties), it's a special pleasure to wade in the lake and watch the sun set over the western mountains.

The landscapes of both the New York and California shelters are beautiful, but in different ways. Summer in Orland means dry, brown grass. Winters can be wet and quite cool, with wind and driving rain. That's when the grass turns a lush green and moves in waves in the wind. In Watkins Glen, hedgerows separate the fields, and there are apple trees and rolling green hills. In autumn the leaves on the trees turn rich shades of red and yellow, while in winter the ground is blanketed in snow and the bare trees are etched against the skyline.

The Orland shelter has a visitors' center with an outdoor pavilion, an overnight cabin, and just as in Watkins Glen, we make the facility available to people who'd like to get married or plan other special events at the farm. We provide lists of vegan-friendly caterers in the area and recommend a bakery nearby that makes terrific vegan wedding cakes.

Like Watkins Glen, Orland is not too far (twenty miles) from a college town, Chico, home to one of California's state universities. Like Cornell, Cal State Chico is an agricultural college, and we often take our interns and volunteers there to expose them to what young farmers are being taught. Chico, similar to Ithaca, has cultural activities and vegetarian restaurants, which provide a nice complement to farm life.

In Orland, as in Watkins Glen, we've built barns and shelters where the animals can come and go as they please except when, in the case of the farmed birds, they need to be protected from coyotes or other predators. There are waterholes for the pigs, ponds for the ducks and geese, perches and roosting areas for the hens, and expansive hillside pastures for grazing. Pigs, sheep, goats, chickens, turkeys, rabbits, ducks, geese, and cattle, all rescued from cruel conditions, make their home at the Orland farm. Both the California and New York shelters house cattle, although different breeds. In parts of the West and throughout the warmer climates, cattle ranchers have been breeding Brahman cattle, originally from India and able to withstand hot climates, with other cattle so they are better able to tolerate the heat. Mixing Angus with Brahman, for example, results in what are called "Brangus" cattle. California also has some Jersey dairy production, and the population of our Orland herd reflects that.

Unique to the California sanctuary are a few donkeys. They weren't farm animals but rather an exotic species introduced to Death Valley National Park, on California's border with Nevada. When the park determined that the donkeys were upsetting the natural ecological balance and decided to cull them, Farm Sanctuary and other sanctuaries agreed to adopt them. The donkeys are well adapted to the dry California climate and spend much of their time in the hills with the cows, sheep, and goats. We also have herds of feral sheep rescued from Santa Cruz Island, off the coast of southern California. They, too, were targeted for extermination. Irresponsible ranchers had left them in a habitat where they didn't belong, and, as often happens, it was the animals who were going to pay the price.

In both shelters, the domestic animals and wild ones occasionally interact. The area surrounding the properties is home to deer, wild turkeys, ducks, and geese who occasionally visit their farmed cousins. In California we now routinely sterilize our sows because the wild pigs are so fond of them. Our California cows are spayed as well. In this case they were the forward ones, paying visits to the beef bulls on neighboring farms. (A bull is a male who has not, like a steer, been neutered.) Occasionally, we also have to spay mature female pigs in Watkins Glen, because when they go into heat they become agitated and frustrated and this causes problems within the herds. All our male mammals are neutered to minimize aggression and potential impregnation.

It's not ideal to curtail the animals' natural impulses to reproduce and raise their young, but the truth is it's the only responsible choice. There are already billions of farmed animals, and we need all the room we can get at the shelters. On rare occasions we have taken in a pregnant animal—usually we don't realize it at first—so a few of the animals in Orland and Watkins Glen have been born there.

Advocacy, West Coast Style

One of the first things we did after the California shelter was up and running was campaign for a state law to prevent the marketing and slaughter of downed animals. Our efforts to move national legislation through Congress failed, but we thought it might be possible to pass legislation state by state. This approach would be more time-consuming and laborious, but we believed we could succeed, and passing state laws could eventually help advance federal legislation.

It made sense to start the effort in California; the dairy industry is the biggest source of downed cows, and California is the country's largest dairy state, with numerous intensive production facilities that push their cows very hard. We began to gather evidence to show the need for legislation. I documented downed cows, animals left to suffer, all over the Golden State. I also located slaughterhouses that specialized in downed animals, as well as dealers who ran operations called cow services. The dealers visited dairy facilities on a daily basis to pick up downed cows and deliver them to these particular slaughterhouses. I witnessed a number of awful scenes at these facilities.

At one slaughterhouse in Modesto, for instance, I stood behind a rendering truck and videotaped cows being shoved with forklifts as if they were pieces of furniture. Another was run as well as any such operation could be. The line speed for the workers wasn't too quick, and the facility had a captive bolt gun to stun the animals, mostly cows, before they were killed. During the course of videotaping the operation and speaking with people on-site, I chatted with a man whom I guessed was in his seventies.

"So, you're an animal person?" he asked.

"Yeah," I replied.

"Are you a vegetarian?" he inquired.

"Uh-huh," I said again.

"Did you read those James Herriot books?" he asked, referring to the popular series written by the English veterinarian. I was surprised we were still talking to each other. Normally the conversation ends abruptly or otherwise disintegrates when slaughterhouse workers hear that I don't eat animals.

"No," I answered. "Have you?"

"Yeah," he replied. "I'm a vegetarian." My mouth fell open. A vegetarian working in a slaughterhouse!

I was so astounded I didn't know what else to say. I later learned from the facility's owner that this man was his mentor. I wondered whether he had worked in the business for a long time and now, reflecting back on his life, had decided he didn't want to eat animals anymore. I suppose he'd asked me if I was a vegetarian to find out if I walked the talk. (People ask me that question all the time.) Strange as it was to find a vegetarian at a slaughterhouse, I took it as a good sign: we all have the power to change, no matter what the circumstances.

Such a pleasant exchange was rare. I remember one visit to a stockyard where I came across a cow too sick to stand. She'd been left in the parking lot and was bellowing in pain. I first spotted her at around three o'clock in the afternoon. I moved on, visiting other stockyards and slaughterhouses, but I couldn't stop thinking about this animal and wondering whether she'd been put out of her misery or not. That evening I went back and found her unmoved and untended to. I called the police, and they answered the call around ten o'clock that night. They spoke with the stockyard manager, then informed me that the cow would to be taken to slaughter the following day. She couldn't be euthanized, he'd explained to the officers, because the cow had to arrive at the slaughterhouse alive in order to be acceptable for use as human food. In short, the officers said, there was nothing they could do to relieve her suffering. Like so many thousands of other downed animals in California and around the United States—creatures too sick or lame to even walk to their own death—this cow was made to endure prolonged pain and fear so the meat on her body could be sold for human consumption. All that suffering for a few dollars.

This incident, and many others like it, formed the evidence that we took to California lawmakers and the media. One state senator, David Roberti, saw the need for a state law on downers and in 1993 introduced legislation to prohibit the slaughter and marketing of downed animals and require them to be humanely euthanized. Farm Sanctuary whole-heartedly supported the effort through public education about the law and the larger issue of downers. The dairy and beef industries put up intense opposition, but we did have the support of Dr. Jim Reynolds, a dairy veterinarian concerned about animal welfare who, for his support of the bill, faced considerable criticism from the industry.

Unlike the national legislation, the effort in California succeeded. The measure, creating California penal code section 599f, was approved by both houses of the legislature and signed by the governor in 1994. It was the first U.S. law to prohibit the marketing and slaughter of downed animals. It was a terrific victory. We hoped it would give momentum to other state-level legislation as well as generate new support in Congress for the Federal Downed Animal Protection Act. Since its passage, 599f has helped prevent the suffering of thousands of downed cows.

The law provides an important legal precedent, and it has resulted in two prosecutions so far. In one, a stockyard manager "euthanized" a calf by hitting him over the head, first with a wooden cane, then with a hammer. The manager pled no contest to charges of improperly killing the calf and was fined and fired. The second case involved a stockyard near Bakersfield where I videotaped downed cows being dragged onto a truck in clear violation of the law. As I was taping, the stockyard manager drove up to my car in a golf cart and told me to leave the property—and I did. I left the parking lot and pulled over on the side of the road. I had with me a copy of the relevant section of the penal code that I wanted to give to the manager. As I was locking my car to return to the stockyard, he appeared in his golf cart.

"Didn't I tell you to leave?" he yelled.

"I did," I replied. "I'm now on a public street."

"This street's my property," he shouted.

I tried to draw his attention to the dragging of cows onto the slaughterhouse truck and offered him the law's text.

"I don't follow that law," he snapped. "I follow the old law. Now, if you don't leave, I'm gonna break your jaw."

As I was getting into my car to leave, the manager hit me in the back with his cattle prod, giving me just a taste of what he and others in the stockyard routinely did to the animals. I made a beeline to the local sheriff's office and returned to the stockyard with an officer. She informed the manager about the law, and in the prosecution that followed he pled guilty. While I can't excuse his actions, I recognize where the impulse to hit me came from—a stockyard is a violent place, and hitting is simply a way of doing business.

At another stockyard I found an unattended downed cow left in the parking lot and began videotaping the scene. When the manager saw what was going on, he approached me, looking angry and swinging a shovel. I was preparing for another confrontation when the police came. The first officer to arrive knew the stockyard manager, and the two men greeted each other warmly. The officer told me he had discretion over whether to issue a citation to the stockyard for violating the law, just as traffic cops can decide whether or not to issue a speeding ticket after pulling somebody over.

He didn't, he said, intend to enforce the law. I rarely, if ever, got off on a speeding charge, I told him. The stockyard was in clear violation of the law, and the officer should issue a citation unless the cow was immediately euthanized or given necessary veterinary attention, I said. Despite my best efforts, I wasn't persuading him. A higher-ranking officer appeared on the scene, one with a more serious view of his law enforcement duties, and asked me for the text of the law. I also offered him a look at the video I'd been shooting—the stockyard manager spewing profanity, approaching my car, waving his shovel overhead, then measuring up a headlight and preparing to smash it. The officer sighed and told me he'd take care of the cow. Within minutes, I heard a gunshot, and the cow was put out of her misery. Somehow that's considered humane euthanasia for farm animals.

Even though we had a good new law on the books in California, it wasn't enough to protect downed animals. We still had work to do to make sure law enforcement officials and the livestock industry knew about the law and abided by it. In the decade since the law passed, we've been visiting stockyards and slaughterhouses to ensure that those working in the industry do comply, and we welcome volunteers who want to help.

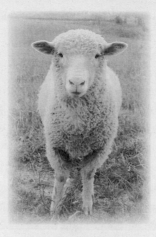

Grace

PROFILE: GRACE

While many of the approximately six million sheep raised for meat or wool in the United States are kept on pasture land, an increasing number are being raised in factory farm feedlots (huge, crowded outdoor enclosures without pasture) or other confinement systems designed to maximize profitability. Whether on pasture or in feedlots, these fragile animals are subjected to sweltering heat in the summer and freezing cold in the winter. In confinement, they live with the stress of crowding. In the United States, the sheep industry's primary salable product is lamb. Approximately four to five million lambs under the age of six months are killed annually, a large percentage around springtime for ethnic and religious holidays. In addition to lambs, thousands of older sheep, mostly ewes past their reproductive prime, are slaughtered each year.

Even in the production of wool, cruelty is a feature. To reduce problems with flies that infest the folds in the skin of Merino sheep (the most highly prized wool breed), producers practice "mulesing." Strips of flesh are literally cut off the backs of the animals' legs and hind region to create smooth skin without anesthesia or pain relievers. Sheep also commonly have their tails cut off to control fly problems.

Grace, a sheep living at the Watkins Glen shelter, managed to escape the fate of most lambs and sheep. She's one of the few animals born at Farm Sanctuary. We don't allow the animals to breed and reproduce (we feel there are far too many unwanted and abused farmed animals already), but Grace's mother came to the shelter along with several other sheep from a farm in Pennsylvania. After the farmer and his wife got to know and appreciate sheep as individuals, they decided they couldn't slaughter their flock. They gave all of them to a shelter in Pennsylvania, which asked us to take in nine of the sheep. When they arrived, we found out that six were pregnant. Our sheep barn was quickly transformed into a maternity ward. By the end of 2004, we'd welcomed eleven new lambs into the world, including Grace and her sister, Dore. Both were born prematurely and were very thin, but thanks to Olive, their protective mother, they thrived.

Now a full-grown ewe, Grace has become quite a star, photogenic and sweet-natured—you can see the kindness in her face. Grace's photo was used on the front cover of Farm Sanctuary's twentieth-anniversary brochure. Ewes remain close to their offspring all their lives, and if they're separated, they'll cry for each other all day. Of all the animals at Farm Sanctuary, sheep probably need each other the most. They're very accepting, and for the most part they can't stand to be alone. Sheep are shy and, well, sheepish, but they're also very curious. Despite what most sheep at Farm Sanctuary have been through, they love people and are fascinated by visitors, even if they don't run up and greet you. When they hear the voices of the staff they recognize at the shelter, they start bleating their hellos.

Sheep usually live for about ten years, although in Watkins Glen a few of the herd are thirteen and older. After many years of grazing, the older sheep lose most of their teeth, and eating grass becomes a challenge. We put them in a separate herd so they don't have to compete with the younger sheep for the best morsels. They also get grain to eat every day. In the warm months, all the sheep at the shelters have to be sheared. Because they've been bred to grow thick coats, they would overheat if they weren't sheared. The sheep don't enjoy the process, but they couldn't be happier to get rid of all that wool in the hot weather.

PART TWO

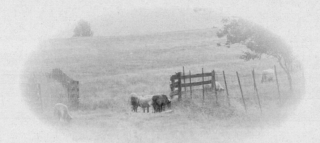

GET BIG

OR

GET OUT

CHAPTER SIX

What's Wrong with the Factory Farm Today

Y ou want to put my people out of business, don't you?"
Those were the words that greeted me when I entered the office of the manager of the swine unit at the University of Florida in Gainesville. He knew I was there to work on a 2002 state ballot initiative that would ban the confinement of female pigs in two-foot-wide gestation crates. The sows (as female pigs are called) are unable to walk or lie down comfortably, and in some cases they remain in crates their whole lives. They experience numerous physical ailments because they have so little space, and show signs of what can only be called insanity, stemming from boredom or extreme frustration.

During my time in Florida, I visited with a number of pork industry representatives, documented the conditions of pigs raised for food in the state, and met many times with volunteers from Floridians for Humane Farms, the coalition group sponsoring the ballot initiative. As part of my work, I arranged a meeting with the swine unit manager. The purpose of his unit, like others in colleges and universities around the country, is to help the animal agriculture industry be more efficient as well as more profitable. Units such as these helped develop many of the practices and systems that are now mainstays of factory farming.

"We don't want to cause anybody harm," I told him, settling into a chair. "We want to prevent suffering. I think it's better for farmers not to be using these kinds of systems, which turn farm work into factory work and animals into production units." He looked skeptical as I made my case that when a pig is in a crate she can't express her normal behaviors.

She can't root in the soil or cool herself in the mud. She can't socialize with other pigs or even her own piglets. She can't even turn around. "She can't be who she is," I concluded.

The manager knew as well as I did that breeding sows' lives are a constant cycle of impregnation, giving birth, and reimpregnation. The only time they are able to walk is when they are moved from one crate to another, or when they are loaded onto trucks to be taken to slaughter. Each of the roughly six million breeding sows in the United States is expected to give birth to two litters a year, or a total of about twenty piglets. Over the course of their lives, breeding sows are fed the barest minimum, only about half of what they would normally eat, and are chronically hungry. Genetically selected to produce fast-growing piglets, the sows, like their offspring, are predisposed to have a strong appetite, which makes their feed restriction even more frustrating.

The manager coolly explained why it was better for the industry, and the sows themselves, to be in the crates. It was also efficient, he said, since crates made it easy to feed the sows and remove their wastes. It was safer, he continued, since the crates protected the pigs from each other and from the elements. It was also, he added, the only practical solution: "I used to raise pigs outside. There are a couple of farmers that do that now, but they're not going to survive. They're going to go out of business. So you have to go to this [confinement] method."

As the manager laid out all the usual arguments for me, I tried to listen respectfully, even though I'd heard the industry's story a hundred times before. To stay in business these days, you have to do A, B, and C. If you don't, you won't make it. For the manager and the agribusiness leaders, the farming extension agents, the economists and animal scientists, farming is a volume business where quantity, not quality, counts. You draw a graph on a computer that shows that if you put this much in and sell at this price, you get this much out. With a volume business, profit margins are smaller. So if you cut costs, you increase profits. And if you make the whole system bigger, you make more. If you don't, you won't—and you'll probably have to close up shop. This is very much like the model Wal-Mart has perfected, the one emptying main streets of small businesses around the country.

It's also just as the late Ruth Harrison, author of the 1964 book *Animal*

Machines, the first exposé of the realities of factory farming, described: "If one person is unkind to an animal, it is considered to be cruelty, but where a lot of people are unkind to animals, especially in the name of commerce, the cruelty is condoned and, once sums of money are at stake, will be defended to the last by otherwise intelligent people."

The swine unit manager's point of view could not be more different from Harrison's and Farm Sanctuary's. To our assertions that animals are not being treated well and the entire system is cruel and inefficient, industry folks such as the manager reply, "What do you mean? We take care of these animals every day." They assume that because they feed and raise so many animals, they understand them. Our perspective is the opposite: you can't get to know animals when they are crammed in two-foot-wide cages, unable to behave normally. The animals are treated badly and the connection between the farmers and the animals is lost. "These animals aren't able to be who they are," I repeated to the manager.

Then something happened. He continued delivering the company line, but it was as if he'd begun (perhaps for the first time) to really listen to what he was saying. He wasn't simply repeating the talking points that corporate public relations specialists provide to agribusiness proponents with the same conviction. His tone had been smug and combative, but now he spoke slowly and deliberately. "You know what's missing today on the farm?" he asked. Without pausing to let me answer, he declared emphatically, "Pigmanship."

Pigmanship. I've since thought a lot about the term and what it might mean. It might mean good animal husbandry, the skillful understanding of an animal, one fostered over generations of farmers. It might mean professionalism, the application of information known to dedicated agriculturalists that allows you to understand the animals, their behavior, and their relationship to the land, so you get the outcomes you want without extreme manipulation. It might just mean a certain decency of behavior, a quiet respect for the interests and characteristics of the pigs in your care. It might be a combination of all of these.

Whatever the manager meant (we didn't discuss it further), I think we both knew that pigmanship—however you define it—is not just missing from today's factory farms, it's actively scorned. Like other farmed animals, pigs are manipulated with feed and living conditions to meet certain growth-rate targets and attain certain market specifications for the slaughterhouse. Every pig now has to be as much like every other pig as possible. Pigmanship has no place on today's industrial farms. Its loss has not just affected pigs; it has drastically changed the welfare of all farmed animals.

A few months later I told the story of my conversation with the swine unit manager during a panel discussion on laws at a bar association meeting in New York City. One of the other panelists, Dr. Paul Sundberg of the National Pork Board, agreed that pigmanship *is* absent from today's farms. I consider both interactions breakthroughs. They suggest to me that in the future there may be room for common ground.

The Real Cost of Cheap Food

The history of industrial development—whatever the industry—tends to follow a pattern. At the birth of a particular industry, competition between early entrants in the market encourages innovation. A few enterprises move ahead of the pack, often by joining with or buying out their competitors and thereby dominating the marketplace. These corporations then consolidate their power and work to stifle competition—say, by controlling prices—as much as they legally can. At the same time, they lobby to prevent or slow government regulation that limits their profitability, while advancing legislation beneficial to their bottom line. Industry leaders curry favor and influence lawmakers, directly or indirectly, through personal gifts, campaign contributions, promises of seats on company boards after they've left office, or threats to move jobs outside legislators' districts. The more they ingratiate themselves with politicians, the more preferential treatment they get.

In this way, the dance of big industry and government continues, often at the expense of smaller businesses and the taxpayer. Perhaps nowhere has this pattern of industrial growth and consolidation been more closely followed than in animal agriculture. That's why it's perhaps fitting that government giveaways for pet projects are called pork.

Farming interests are continuously seeking more money from the government. Agriculturalists use the phrase *farming the government* to describe the process, and a lot of corporate farmers obviously spend more time in Washington, D.C., lobbying for federal money than they do on the land. Federal subsidies or farm aid totaled $25 billion in 2005, including some $1.3 billion that went to people who weren't even farmers but only lived on land that used to be farmed. Most of this federal money went not to small family farmers but to large operations, many of which are controlled by even larger corporations. According to a 2006 report prepared by the Environmental Working Group, fifty-four entities, most of them substantial, collected farm aid in the form of subsidies averaging more than $100,000. By contrast, more than 300,000 smaller farms received only a pittance, less than $100. The federal government also continues to provide subsidies to corporate farming for expanding operations, including systems to manage waste from confined animals.

Other government actions have enabled the consolidation and intensification of animal agriculture since World War II. Laws preventing businesses from merging and acquiring each other have been relaxed, and today a handful of companies dominate the marketplace for animal products. In addition, subsidies have aided the production of enormous amounts of cheap corn, soybeans, and other crops for farm animal feed. According to the Institute for Agriculture and Trade Policy, between 2000 and 2004 an average of $4.5 billion a year in federal subsidies went to support corn production. Around 60 percent of the corn produced in the United States is used to feed farmed animals. Low prices and a massive supply of corn and soybeans have contributed to a shift away from grass as a major feed source and have made it efficient to confine and feed massive numbers of animals indoors.

This consolidation has taken place at the same time as, and as a result of, the emergence of consumer culture in the 1950s and 1960s. The production of automobiles on a massive scale, cheap oil, and the extension of the interstate highway system across the country all fueled the trend. The growing fast-food industry demanded cheap food and predictability of products so that a McDonald's hamburger, for instance, would taste the same in Duluth as it did in San Diego.

Federal and state departments of agriculture and land grant universities have also played a role in helping industry to produce large numbers of animals more efficiently. The land grant university system was established in 1862 under President Lincoln. The federal government gave each state ten thousand acres of land to establish public universities that would teach agriculture and engineering. Other universities, both public and private, have also established colleges or departments of agriculture and life sciences.

Land grant colleges were designed to support agricultural research and education. The long-term goal was to ensure a plentiful and safe supply of food. In time, however, the arrival of big business on campuses has compromised the integrity of academic institutions focused on agriculture, no less than it has in other fields. These public and private institutions have helped agribusiness to develop the chemical additives and industrialized production methods in use today. They have also assisted with genetic innovations. Selective breeding has created animal "units" that produce under the stresses of confinement and grow to the specifications set by industry. It worked in some ways—these methods do shave dollars and increase production—but as I've demonstrated in previous chapters, the costs have simply been moved elsewhere.

For starters, the taxes we pay fund the agribusiness subsidies; we pay more for health care because of our blood pressure and cholesterol readings; our property values collapse when a factory farm relocates nearby. Our environment, too, has suffered. We have denuded the countryside not only of farmed animals but also of other fauna and flora as we have turned complex and diverse ecosystems into monoculture feed crops that stretch as far as the eye can see. We have removed manure as a source of soil nutrients and replaced it with petrochemical fertilizers, increasing our dependence on oil while polluting our streams and killing aquatic life in our rivers and oceans. Likewise, waste and wastewater from concentrated animal feeding operations are fouling rivers, streams, and coastal waters.

We are draining or diverting rivers and aquifers by raising animals and growing crops where we shouldn't be to meet the industry's seemingly relentless demand for resources. Large slaughterhouses that kill cattle use between 250,000 and 500,000 gallons of water each day. Poultry plants use even more, about 1.5 million gallons per day (about 6 gallons per bird). The Ogallala aquifer, which lies under 175,000 square miles and eight states in the High Plains, has been a repository of fresh water for millions of years. "The trouble is," as *Drovers,* an industry journal, reports, "the aquifer is running dry—seriously dry. And for an industry such as food production that relies on water not just to grow crops and livestock but also to keep operations sanitized and food clean, running out of water means running out of business."

It is true that everyone in the industrialized world, and increasingly around the globe, today has more access to farmed animal products than ever before. Indeed, so many of us live "high on the hog" and enjoy the fat of the land that it's not surprising that we have never been heavier. In 2005, for instance, each American ate a record high amount of meat and poultry—nearly 190 pounds. Currently, 64.5 percent of U.S. adults age twenty and older are overweight, and 30.5 percent are obese. Globally, the World Health Organization estimates, more than 1 billion people are overweight—while, tragically, nearly 850 million more are chronically hungry. We pack on the pounds in affluent cultures in a manner that rather perversely parallels the animals we eat, who have been bred to grow big, fast—until both eater and eaten can no longer function normally and begin to suffer health problems.

We pay the price for farm consolidation in others ways, too. No one really knows why, but antibiotics make farmed animals grow faster. This has resulted in agribusiness using a phenomenal twenty-five million pounds a year—that's *eight times* the amount used to treat human illnesses. We are increasingly making ourselves vulnerable to bacterial infections that develop immunity to normal lines of antibiotic treatment. Hormones in animal products have been linked to the ever-younger ages at which boys and girls reach puberty. Then there are mad cow disease, pfiesteria, salmonella, campylobacter, *E. coli,* and other potentially fatal pathogens that flourish in the fecal stew of the feedlots, factory farms, and slaughterhouses. Add to that the public health risks of respiratory and neurological disease, cancer, and depression. Given these facts, it's not that much of a stretch to say that our health care crisis is closely tied to the health crisis in the animal agriculture industry.

It's also no secret that factory farm operations and slaughterhouses exploit a low-paid, expendable labor force with little power to challenge their dismal working or living conditions. Wherever it sets up shop, industrial agriculture seems to breed a number of social sicknesses—

desperation, alienation, alcoholism, spousal abuse, and other violent crimes that destroy families and communities. As the editors of *Any Way You Cut It: Meat Processing in Small-Town America* explain, communities that attract processing plants "can also expect to be confronted with school overcrowding, homelessness, housing shortages, elevated unemployment, crime, and social disorders." Instead of turning swords into plowshares, the industrialization of agriculture has resulted in violence, corruption, cruelty, and pollution, and we ingest it at every meal.

Modern Serfdom

As corporate control over agriculture has intensified, many farmers have become contract growers. This term obscures the reality that for many it's a form of modern serfdom. The farmer assumes the risks, but the corporation owns the collateral. If a farmer, for instance, wants to raise pigs or chickens, he will have to conform to the industry or corporation's production requirements. This means constructing sheds and structures to the company's specifications. Building these facilities isn't cheap, so while there may be subsidies to help, the farmer typically needs to take out loans, or several loans. To make a living, he has to raise a lot of animals and meet production targets tied to the square footage of his facility.

While the large-volume producers have the wherewithal to survive short-term losses and capital to bolster production and maintain profit margins, small contract growers are less secure when they fall behind their production targets. When they do, their pay is less, and given this loss of expected income, they may not be able to make their payments to the bank. They can lose everything. Remember, it's the farmer who assumes all the liabilities. He or she pays for the materials and the labor to put up the building, look after the animals, dispose of their waste, and maintain the operation to the corporation's specifications. The farmer takes the fall if the enterprise falters or fails. From the standpoint of profit making for the corporation, it's a brilliant model.

Arkansas-based Tyson, which calls itself the "world's largest processor and marketer of chicken, beef, and pork," has thousands of contract growers. Like many so-called integrators, Tyson is so big that the power it wields over contract farmers is immense. "I am a slave to Tyson," one grower explained in Steve Striffler's book *Chicken: The Dangerous Transformation of America's Favorite Food.* I've heard words to that effect many times myself. "Tyson is the only game in town. It's the integrator around here so there is no choice, no competition. If Tyson wants improvements, you make them, you pay for them, and you smile real nice. And in exchange, if you keep your mouth shut and work hard, you keep getting chicks delivered so you can pay the mortgage." If Tyson decides one grower's animals aren't to its specifications, it can refuse to buy them, potentially leaving the farmer with thousands of animals and nowhere to sell them. If Tyson wants to shift production from one contractor to another, it can move its business out, just like that. The grower is left with the shed, loan payments, and often a huge mess of manure and animal carcasses to clean up. Needless to say, the result can be dreadful for the farmer and the animals.

Several years ago in Alabama, a contract grower for Tyson was throwing dead chickens from his facility into a pit on his property. When it began overflowing, he took the dead chickens to the local dump. It turned out some of them weren't dead—the farmer just wanted to get rid of them. One of our members called and said that she was running around the dump picking up live chickens! Some of the rescued birds ended up at our Watkins Glen shelter.

The "get bigger or get out" mantra embraced by economists, corporate agribusiness titans, and land grant universities means that the farmers push their animals very hard to get the levels of production the spreadsheet demands—and many still can't do it. For farm families who have proudly maintained their land for generations, debt-free and independent, the demands of modern farming can be too much. For decades, we've seen the foreclosure and death of thousands of family farms. A few years ago, Brian Halweil of the Worldwatch Institute calculated that there are now more prisoners than farmers in the United States. Sometimes it's hard to tell the difference.

When I visit rural communities, I often see discontent, alienation, and depression. Farmers are scared. "How can I make a living?" they ask. "I know how to farm. My family has been farming for generations. But with this new model, it's impossible." Farmers almost universally complain about how hard things are and how saddened they are to see their children leave the farm because they just can't make a living.

I think one of the reasons why industrial farmers get so angry at people like me is that they know at some level that what they are doing is wrong and that this kind of "farming" has lost its honor. They don't want to be confronted with their own doubts. In an industrial pig operation, for instance, the farmer manages what is in essence a factory. Workers check on feeding and watering equipment and temperature control mechanisms, and use high-speed water systems to hose down the pigs' feces and wash it away into massive slurries. The farmer is a technician monitoring charts and following a production blueprint in a quasi-laboratory—a far cry from pigmanship. It is also perhaps why the suicide rate among farmers and ranchers in the United States is now three times higher than the national average.

Breeding Disease

As part of a court case, one of the lawyers who volunteers her time with Farm Sanctuary, Melissa Bonfiglio, and I were allowed to visit a pig production facility as part of what is called the discovery (fact-gathering) process of a court case. Legally I'm not allowed to describe what I saw there, but I can tell you what we had to go through before we even *entered* the facility. We were asked to undress and then go into a shower stall and wash with antimicrobial soap and shampoo. After that, we moved to another stall and put on the facility's coveralls and boots so our bodies were completely covered. When we left, we reversed the process, removing our full-body suits and showering again. Only then could we put on our civilian clothes and go back outdoors. It was similar to the process you'd have to go through to enter or leave a biohazard site.

The fear, of course, was that we might be carrying pathogens that could sicken all the animals in the building. Because animals bred for food today have very little genetic diversity and are crowded so closely together indoors, their natural resistance to infections has been eroded.

If one virus gets loose, it could destroy a whole herd. Even if a virus is far from fatal, it could harm productivity by reducing fertility so that the sows, for instance, wouldn't continue to breed or would have fewer piglets in each litter. Maintaining disease-free herds is critical to modern farm economics. If you're in a state or country where a particular animal disease is known to exist, you may be prevented from selling to other states or countries that are free of the disease. So diseases can mean substantial losses even if the disease is not fatal to the animal.

In 2001 foot-and-mouth disease (also known as hoof-and-mouth) was found on English farms. Soon the disease was identified in other parts of Britain, and whole areas of England, Wales, Scotland, and Northern Ireland were cordoned off as hundreds of farmers were instructed by the government to kill all their animals as a preventive measure, even if they showed no signs of the disease. Huge pyres were built to burn the bodies. The aim was to "eradicate" foot-and-mouth so that the United Kingdom could resume selling its animals to other disease-free countries. Although only two thousand confirmed cases of foot-and-mouth were ever documented, about six *million* farm animals were killed. And it's still unlikely the disease will ever be totally eradicated.

A similar series of events unfolded when mad cow disease was discovered in the herds of several countries. The United States stopped importing their beef, arguing that it didn't want the disease in this country. However, when mad cow disease was discovered in the United States in December 2003 (additional cases have now been confirmed, but they appear to be of an "atypical" strain; some industry watchers believe mad cow is more widespread than reported) and countries started banning imports of our meat, our trade representatives fought mightily to convince foreign markets to take our beef.

Most Americans assume that government agencies are working to safeguard our citizens from disease and bad food. Theoretically, they're right. When President Lincoln established the USDA in the 1860s to provide advice and support for the agrarian community, he called it the "people's department." But it seems to have lost its way, and now it often serves the interests of industrial farmers, at the expense of traditional family farmers and society at large. The USDA's current mandate is to promote the business of agriculture, which can be in direct conflict with its mandate to protect human health. Over many years, senior officials of the USDA have either come from or moved on to jobs in agribusiness, creating at the very least a perception of a revolving door of influence.

The result is a regrettable don't-ask-don't-tell policy when it comes to food safety. The public doesn't get adequate information from the USDA about the food supply, and when a disease does break out, such as *E. coli* or salmonella, consumers are blamed for not preparing or cooking food properly, while the industry usually escapes government censure. If the U.S. government and the farmed animal industry were genuinely concerned about disease in farmed animals, we would test more rigorously for BSE and Johne's disease (a wasting condition that affects the intestinal system of cattle) and other pathogens. We wouldn't let downed animals enter the food chain. We wouldn't feed animals huge amounts of antibiotics as a standard part of their diet. We wouldn't reduce the genetic diversity of farmed animals. And we wouldn't confine animals in overcrowded, stressful conditions, which exacerbate the spread of disease.

Whatever the immediate cause of a food-borne illness, we still aren't addressing how and why these pathogens are created and spread in the first place. As Upton Sinclair wrote, in a passage Al Gore harked back to for his Academy Award–winning documentary *An Inconvenient Truth:* "It is difficult to get a man to understand something when his salary depends on his not understanding it."

The California pig facility we visited as a prelude to the court case I mentioned above illustrates a larger point about the senselessness of our current farming practices. When you think of what it means to be a farmer, you probably think of someone in contact with nature's rhythms and cycles, a custodian of an ancient knowledge about the land and the seasons. People imagine rich loam, the sweet smell of hay, and a palmful of seeds. We picture healthy farm animals grazing the land and resting inside warm, hay-filled barns when it's cold or stormy. We know farming is a tough, physical life, but the work is honest and has rewards that extend beyond money alone. It is work done in the service of feeding people *and* tending the land, productive not only for the farmer but also for his or her family and the larger community over generations. What you're picturing is pigmanship, and it's sadly absent on today's farms.

For factory farmers and their animals, there is no connection with nature or dirt, no experience of the sun or wind or rain or snow. No space is set aside for the animals to root or nest or forage or graze. In fact, in the case of the pig facility we visited, anything to do with the natural world or living organisms, including us, is treated as a hazard. We have the bizarre situation where what's seen as a sophisticated and modern method of producing animals—animal science—is actually more dangerous to the animals and us than the old ways of animal husbandry.

I believe most farmers are good, hardworking people. Most see themselves performing an honorable and necessary service: feeding a hungry world. It's the older generation of farmers, I've found, who lament what's happened. They tell me about a time, in the not-so-distant past, when farmers worked *with* the land and their animals, not against them; a time when farming wasn't reduced to mechanical calculations of inputs and outputs; a time when animals grazed and rooted and pecked in the soil instead of being encased in warehouses where neither sun nor fresh air can reach them. But these things are relics now, from a world that's nearly lost.

What Ralph Nader said all those years ago when I first heard him speak has never rung more true to me. We've become very good at producing and marketing food but not very good at consuming it or recognizing its side effects. We've created mass production at low prices, a system that operates under duress. There are stressed-out pigs who can't mate, who bite one another's tails because they're so confined, or who are so heavy their legs can no longer support their bodies; turkeys who can't reproduce naturally; chickens who have to be debeaked because they peck at each other in densely packed cages; roosters bred for growth who've become so aggressive that they injure or kill their mates; and cows who eat other cows as part of their feed and go mad.

All of this is presided over by stressed-out farmers, many of whom have come to accept the industry's bigger-is-better mantra, though it's clearly unsustainable for them and the earth. In the process they have become almost as trapped as the animals they "farm." Farmers, industry, and consumers have created a treadmill that runs ever more rapidly, fueled by all kinds of suffering animals—including us. It's a system that only takes and doesn't give back; it extracts and doesn't replenish, until the creatures and the earth that sustain its existence have nothing more to give.

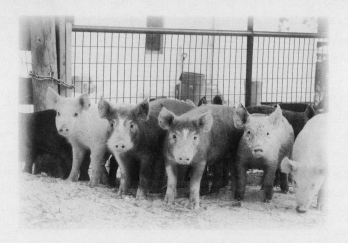

Susie's piglets (and friends)

PROFILE: SUSIE AND HER PIGLETS

In early December 2002, we received a call about 128 pigs and piglets on a farm in Cattaraugus County, New York, living in conditions so terrible that the stunned SPCA officer who found them had to spend more than a few minutes collecting himself before deciding what action to take. The officer had been told that twenty pigs were in distress, so he was understandably alarmed to find six times that number. The farmer, who was subsequently charged with more than a hundred counts of cruelty to animals, had left the pigs to fend for themselves in temperatures that dipped into the single digits, with bitter wind chills that made it feel as cold as thirty below. The water troughs were empty or had frozen over. Some of the pigs huddled to-gether to keep warm; others were skinny and sick; some were literally frozen to the ground and unable to move. Nine of the animals had to be euthanized on the spot, while another five died over the next few days.

Taking in and then adopting so many large animals was a huge, expensive challenge for us. So Farm Sanctuary launched a campaign to help the surviving pigs find good homes—but only after we'd treated them for a range of diseases, including E. coli, stomach bloating, pneu-monia, lung and ear infections, parasites, skin wounds, mange, and ab-scesses. Many of the piglets were red and white or black and white and very cute, so finding homes for them was relatively easy. We worried, though, that potential adopters would be nervous to take in Duroc pigs, a breed that can grow very large (up to nine hundred pounds) and develop leg and foot problems as a result.

For several months some of the pigs were cared for at foster homes, usually farms, while we took care of others at the Watkins Glen shelter. Sadly, nearly fifty more of the pigs died. In the end we found homes for sixty-eight pigs and piglets in places as far-flung as Colorado, Massachu-setts, Michigan, Oklahoma, Texas, Kansas, Florida, and Montana.

Susie was one of the sows rescued from the farm with her piglets Carmen, Cameron, Cody, and Collin. Susie and the piglets were placed in separate pens at a foster farm while we figured out what to do with the smaller and larger male and female pigs. In January 2003, when Farm Sanctuary staff came with an SPCA officer to transport the four piglets to Farm Sanctuary (we weren't able to take Susie at that time), Cameron slipped out of the officer's grasp and ran to his mother's pen. For a good ten minutes we tried to distract Susie, who lunged at any-one who came near. Finally, we succeeded, and the piglets came to Farm Sanctuary.

A month later, Carmen, Cameron, Cody, and Collin were among a group of six piglets adopted by a Farm Sanctuary supporter in Texas. When the supporter heard about Cameron's escape, she resolved to take eight-hundred-pound Susie, too. The farmer who'd been looking after Susie told us that she was aggressive and dangerous, and so when Susie arrived at her new home, we encouraged the adopting family to place her in a pen away from the piglets. The plan was to keep them apart for a couple of weeks and then slowly allow Susie to spend time with the piglets to make sure no one was injured.

The plan didn't last long. The next morning at feeding time, the caretaker was first surprised and then alarmed to find the piglets missing. As she looked more closely, however, she saw a hole next to their pen. When she went over to Susie's pen, she saw another hole and finally the welcome sight of Susie and the four piglets snuggled together in the deep straw. Since then the five of them have been inseparable. What the farmer had taken for Susie's dangerous aggression had really been simply a mother's anguish at having her babies taken away.

CHAPTER SEVEN

The Real Deal on Veal

It was in California that we encountered another unsavory by-product of the dairy industry in its most acute form—vast numbers of unwanted male calves. One of the common misconceptions I've encountered over the years is the notion that if you don't eat meat, you don't contribute to the cruel treatment of animals. "Cows give milk, right?" people ask. "It's natural. That's what they do." What many people don't realize is that cows have to be impregnated to produce milk, and unless the cow miscarries, a calf will be born. If the calf is female, she will likely be raised to produce milk, just like her mother. But if the calf is male, he is essentially useless to the dairy industry: he can't produce milk or give birth to more calves.

After World War II the dairy industry grew dramatically and soon faced a production dilemma. What could be done with all those male calves? The agribusiness answer was veal—in other words, a whole new industry. What happens to the male calves who become veal doesn't make for pleasant reading, but it's an issue that can't be ignored.

Soon after he's born—often within the first few minutes of his life—a male calf is taken from his mother. Many are trucked to stockyards, where veal producers bid on them. I have seen male calves, some barely a day old, prodded into stockyard rings, wobbling on their spindly legs. The calves are presented, their weights announced, and they're auctioned to the highest bidder. Some of the calves are so young that their umbilical cords are still attached. Others, still unsteady on their legs, like Opie, fall at the stockyard and find they can't get up. They are among the youngest downers.

Others go down even before they leave the dairies. Here, their value is so low that they may be sold for rendering or even deposited on the dead pile while they're still alive. That's what happened to Mario, a male Jersey calf rescued by a rendering service truck driver. The driver was so shocked and upset to find a live animal left for dead that he helped get the calf to Farm Sanctuary. Mario was so severely injured that it took five surgeons at the University of California at Davis veterinary school four hours to correct a fracture in his leg. He spent weeks wearing a splint and learning how to walk again, but after several months he could run and buck just like a healthy calf, even with his splint. Now full-grown, Mario lives at our Orland shelter.

If he's not put on the dead pile and survives the journey to the veal operation, whether the calf passes through a stockyard first or is sold directly from the dairy, he'll be housed in a narrow crate—just two feet wide—in an indoor shed. So will hundreds of others like him. Here is where the calf will spend the approximately twenty weeks of his short life. He will be chained by the neck, unable to turn around, and barely able to shift his body. To further discourage the calf from moving, the shed will be kept dark. His all-liquid diet will be low in iron and devoid of fiber, and as a result, he will experience borderline anemia. Production demands dictate these conditions to prevent the calf's flesh from becoming red or muscled. Pallor and tenderness are the qualities prized by some chefs and some diners.

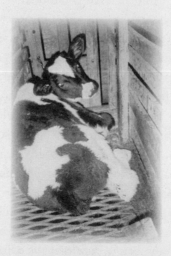

A veal calf in a crate

The calf's close confinement also meets another industry production goal. Instead of burning calories through exercise, more of the calf's caloric intake goes toward putting on pounds—maximizing growth while minimizing feed costs. Since he can barely move, the calf is less likely to injure himself, though it is a real possibility in his weakened state.

I have to shake my head at the "logic" of this system. While this method of rearing calves may be supremely efficient—low expense leading to big income—the unaccounted costs are huge. One is sick animals, including downers. When the calves are sent to slaughter, some can barely walk onto the truck, like a calf I found left in an alleyway at an empty veal facility in upstate New York. Then there are the devastating circumstances of the calves' lives and the human callousness that allows this.

Cows are social animals who ruminate, graze, and spend time together. All of this is denied to veal calves. To cope with the boundaries of their small, hard crates, calves commonly behave in ways animal researchers associate with frustration. They may toss or shake their heads, roll their tongues, and scratch, kick, and lick the walls of their crates. I have been inside veal production facilities and have seen fear, boredom, and despair in the eyes of hundreds of young calves. It is heartrending to see.

Yet even this level of deprivation isn't enough for some producers, who, eager for even more output with even less effort, cut corners. In these facilities, the conditions are even worse—something difficult to imagine unless you've seen it.

At a farm in Wisconsin, a leading veal production state, I found calf after calf standing or lying in their crates, caked in feces and surrounded by flies. The stench was overpowering. In the late 1980s, a Pennsylvania veal farmer became annoyed at the feed company for which he was a contract grower. His contract stated the conditions under which he had to raise the calves, who belonged to the feed company, not him. When there was a dispute about the contract, he took his frustrations with the company out on the calves. One day his neighbors heard the calves bellowing and called the local authorities. They found a barn full of sixty dead and decaying animals. The remaining fifteen or so survivors were emaciated, some with their chains embedded in their necks. The farmer had simply stopped feeding the calves.

The authorities charged the farmer with cruelty and temporarily re-located the calves to a local farm, where they were nursed back to health. Farm Sanctuary was called about the case, and the calves came to live with us on the tofu farm in Pennsylvania; later we adopted most of them out to good homes. The farmer was convicted, a landmark ruling.

A Call for Change

While these are particularly awful cases of neglect, even clean, well-maintained veal farms are inherently problematic because of the indus-try's standard practices. Back in the 1970s, activists began documenting these practices and shared what they learned and saw with the American public. The facts made their way to my grandmother and, through her, to me. What struck home was the image of a young calf separated from his mother and chained in a crate in darkness, unable to move, for the rest of his life. Many women identified with the mother cows who lost their infants. They also felt great compassion for the solitary calves. In the late 1980s, the Mother's Day No Veal Campaign was born.

For years, people have come together in cities and towns across the United States around Mother's Day to raise consciousness about the plight of veal calves. At these gatherings, people hand out informational leaflets to passersby and patrons in front of restaurants and stores that continue to sell veal. Some communities hold candlelight vigils to ac-knowledge the veal calves' suffering and their mothers' losses. In addi-tion, actress Lindsay Wagner, a longtime vegetarian, appeared in a tele-vised public service announcement (PSA) on veal production produced by Farm Sanctuary.

As part of our campaign against crated veal or, "milk-fed veal," as it's also known, we have argued that all calves should be given space to exer-cise, have the ability to interact with other calves and engage in natural behaviors, and be fed a nutritious diet that supports their normal physi-cal development. These public education efforts have had an impact. Increasingly, veal from crated, anemic calves is moving off the plates of caring consumers throughout the United States. Since the launch of the no-veal campaign, veal consumption per person in the United States has dropped from an average of 1.6 pounds a year in 1986 to about half a pound today, a decline of over two-thirds.

We have also reached out to restaurant chefs and managers to make them aware of the cruelty involved in producing veal and urge them to stop selling it. More than four hundred restaurants in twenty-eight states and Washington, D.C., have signed our No Veal Pledge, agreeing not to serve veal from calves raised in crates and fed an anemia-causing diet. Many have dropped veal from their menus entirely.

Some veal producers have come to believe that current production methods need to change, partly because so many consumers will no longer eat the meat. A few farmers have begun to house calves in more spacious environments, sometimes on pasture, and in groups so they can socialize. Some even allow the calves to live with their mothers for a time. Other producers now mix elements of factory and free-range farming. Calves may live in groups, but they are kept indoors on slatted floors. Some veal calves are also living longer—up to twenty-four weeks—as producers develop the technological means to keep their meat white despite the calves' older age. But a slightly longer life doesn't necessarily mean a happier or a healthier one. At the end of their lives these calves are denied as much iron as possible so that when they're slaughtered the flesh is suitably pale.

The industry's large producers have made some changes, and it's only fair to acknowledge them. But it's also only fair to say that these changes are little more than cosmetic. For instance, the sides of the veal crates have been shortened so calves are no longer fully enclosed. Some producers claim that the calves can now turn around, groom themselves, and interact with other calves. Unfortunately, the reality is a little less comforting. The crate, which remains a mere twenty-two inches wide, no longer reaches past the middle of the calf's body. This does allow him to move his rump, but little more. The tether permits the calves to just about lick their shoulders, but they still don't have a full range of movement, and they can't turn around. They can poke their noses through the fronts of their crates and touch each other. They can also lean up against each other through the crate, and tap each other with their hooves. Still, no objective observer would describe these interactions as normal.

The simple truth is that the calves still can't walk or run, play or graze, or feel fresh air, sunlight, or even rain on their backs. Scientists have documented the harmful effects of these unnatural conditions. In research conducted at Texas A&M University in the mid-1980s, animal scientists found crated veal calves showed increased levels of adrenal and thyroid hormones consistent with high levels of stress. The calves also experienced higher illness and mortality rates and needed more medication than their non-crated counterparts. A wealth of studies by European scientists, including the scientific veterinary commission of the European Union, has since corroborated the findings of the Texas A&M study. Owing to this research and public concern about the cruelty involved, most European countries have banned crated veal production altogether.

Even though growing numbers of consumers refuse to eat it, veal has not yet disappeared from American menus. Each year, about seven hundred thousand male calves are slaughtered at about twenty weeks of age and sold as white veal. The veal industry, for the most part, has battened down its hatches instead of adapting to consumer demands and increasingly accepted norms of animal welfare. It's their critics who have the problem, the producers charge, not them.

The industry and its trade groups, such as the American Veal Association, have fought vigorously against legislative proposals that would require calves be fed a healthy diet and given enough space to turn around. They have argued that scientific research has shown that when calves are fed fiber and iron they become sick. They have also claimed that a calf should not suckle from his mother because he could be more susceptible to disease! Industry representatives have even suggested that if a calf were allowed to exercise or turn around he'd be at risk of eating his own feces, and therefore of getting ill.

It's worth delving into these arguments, since they reflect the factory producer's mind-set and the production-at-all-costs credo that has come to dominate animal agriculture. They also show how far industrial farming has strayed from concepts of husbandry and how out of sync it is with who these animals are and what they need.

In natural surroundings, calves start grazing when they are only a few days old. As they nibble on grass, their rumen, a part of the digestive system that will ultimately become a massive stomach, begins to develop.

By six months, it's a fully functioning organ. But if calves are never fed solid food, as is the case with factory-farmed veal calves, they remain "pre-ruminant"—in other words, they don't develop a normal rumen. So it's no surprise they have digestive problems, especially when suddenly fed straw, grass, or other fiber-rich foods.

If he's allowed to, a calf will nurse from his mother perhaps a dozen times a day, drinking a little bit at a time. In this way, he takes in nourishment at a pace his body can handle. In veal facilities, calves are fed a large volume of formula twice a day, distending their young stomachs. This twice-a-day feeding regimen is convenient for veal producers, but it can lead to more difficulties with the calves' digestive organs. In case it's not perfectly clear yet, I'll spell it out: it's the system that is creating the problem, not the calves.

As to the industry's claim that calves should not be allowed to turn around so they don't eat their own wastes, that's an invented problem, too. No calf eats his own waste—unless, perhaps, he's forced to live in a closely confined space. Veal producers want calves lined up in rows, like pieces of machinery, unable to turn around. That way, their excretions fall into the manure collection gutter at the back of their crates. Efficiency is paramount: the calves can be fed at the front and hosed down at the back. The industry tests the calves' blood for iron levels because if they became clinically anemic the calves would stop eating and gaining weight. But the amount of iron the calves get is the bare minimum they need. Borderline anemia doesn't make a healthy calf.

Another little-known practice of the veal industry is its dependence on drugs. We're talking about massive doping. In 2004, a USDA vet in Wisconsin detected a hormone implant in a veal calf. Further investigation revealed that as many as 90 percent of veal calves have been fed a steady diet of synthetic testosterone, though the practice is illegal, and testosterone-fed veal's effects on humans who eat it are unknown. (This growth hormone has been approved for use only in adult cows.) For a time, the USDA stopped veal calves who had been given the synthetic testosterone from entering the food supply. The industry's reaction to public furor was sadly typical—a spokesman for the American Veal Association told *USA Today* that it was much ado about nothing. Growth hormones, he said, had been fed to veal calves for thirty years!

Unfortunately, state and federal legislatures in the United States have failed to enact laws to protect veal calves or regulate the conditions in which they are raised, despite our own and others' efforts. In 2004, Farm Sanctuary worked intensively to get a law passed in New Jersey that would have banned the offensive practices. The bill passed the state senate and was voted out of committee in the assembly, but then died on the assembly floor. It seems that the restaurant industry and pharmaceutical corporations, both of which are quite influential in New Jersey politics, saw the bill as a threat and played a major role in killing it. We'll keep trying. In fact, Farm Sanctuary worked with an alliance of humane organizations in Arizona on a 2006 ballot initiative to ban the use of veal crates. There's more on that to come.

In the Texas A&M study, researchers found that, in addition to the health problems typical of veal calves, they displayed a tendency to run, jump, and socialize with others when released from the crates and the tethers. I'm not surprised. That's what the children of most mammals do.

The Farm Industry Adapts

As the veal industry slowly declines, dairy operators have been searching for other ways to make money from surplus male calves. One idea they have hit upon is changing industry norms about which breeds of cattle are suitable for beef. For many years, farmers assumed that Holsteins— the familiar black and white cows you often see on milk and yogurt cartons—didn't make good beef cattle. As a result, most male Holstein calves ended up in veal production facilities. But in recent years, the conventional wisdom has changed. When I was a student at Cornell in the mid-1990s, scientists were conducting research on Holstein carcasses to test their desirability for beef production. They concluded that the Holsteins, in fact, did make suitable beef cattle.

The industry took notice, and quickly. Just a couple of years after I graduated, I began noticing numerous Holsteins among the traditional breeds on beef feedlots. Feedlots are enormous virtual "cattle cities" where the animals are fattened, mostly on corn, for slaughter. But beef and dairy producers still needed a place to send male calves to grow big and strong enough to join other cattle in the feedlot. So they set up "calf ranches," increasingly common way stations for young calves. With the dominance of the dairy industry in California, it follows that both the number and size of calf ranches in the state are considerable. Some house tens of thousands of calves, both male and female. And transporting newly born calves from dairy farms and to the calf ranches has developed into a big business in California and other parts of the country with large concentrated dairy operations.

Even though the male calves on these "ranches" have escaped the veal crate, their living conditions are far from luxurious and bear little resemblance to what the word *ranch* implies—pasture, nature, and socializing in herds. The "ranch" typically consists of long rows of covered wooden boxes about three feet wide and six feet long, each housing a single calf. Sounds a lot like a veal crate, doesn't it?

For the first couple of months of their lives the calves can't exercise or interact with other calves. While they aren't anemic, the calves are fed milk replacer and antibiotics, to prevent disease. Unlike calves raised for veal, they are also fed grain, a practice that flies in the face of the industry's own argument that solid food is bad for calves. When they're about eight weeks old, the calves are usually placed in a group pen. If they're male, they'll be raised for beef. Females become replacement heifers if they remain healthy and look like they're going to be good milk producers. If they're not and are still below a certain age, they can be slaughtered and sold as veal. Besides the white veal that comes from crated, anemic calves, there are other types of veal, including "bob" veal, which comes from young calves—less than three weeks old and sometimes as young as a day or two. Calves killed for bob veal sell for less, and their meat is used in less expensive products such as TV dinners.

Calf ranches haven't changed the fundamental economics that make male calves in the dairy industry disposable, and downed calves still aren't uncommon at slaughterhouses and on calf ranches. What *is* new is that a somewhat freer market has developed for the male calves. They are potentially useful to the beef industry, and their fate isn't necessarily a short, miserable life spent in a crate. But their value fluctuates wildly in the marketplace and can drop very low. Newborn male calves, especially those who are sick, may earn only a few dollars at stockyards, so sellers are often desperate to get rid of them any way they can.

Small Victories

The market that has developed in the industry around male calves can resemble the Wild West. It's governed by few rules, and there's little industry accountability and plenty of room for cruelty.

In 1999, on a typically hot August day in Phoenix, Arizona, two police officers pulled over the driver of a battered blue Chevy Impala with no license plates. As the two officers questioned the driver, they heard pounding noises coming from the trunk. When they opened it, they were stunned to find six two-day-old Jersey calves hog-tied—their front and hind legs roped together—and covered in their own waste. By the officers' estimation it was 110 degrees outside, making it considerably hotter inside that trunk. The officers took the calves to the Arizona Humane Society. A vet on staff diagnosed the calves as severely dehydrated and near death.

The Arizona Humane Society did not typically take in and treat farm animals, and it wasn't set up to care for this kind of domestic animal. Luckily, one of the staff members had grown up on a farm and knew what to do with the Jerseys, who, with their doelike eyes and soft brown skin, look just like fawns. She cooled the calves down by rubbing them with alcohol, then gave them fluids through an IV as well as colostrum (calves' first food from their mothers) to boost their immune system. The calves suckled hungrily on oversized bottles of milk.

Over the next four days, the shelter staff adjusted their schedules to ensure that the calves had twenty-four-hour care. Sadly, despite all their hard work, two of the calves died. The condition of the other four went up and down, but eventually it stabilized. When they were strong enough, the shelter arranged for them to live with a longtime friend of the Arizona Humane Society who had a large backyard and could foster the calves. In the meantime, the staff searched for permanent homes. These four little guys, after surviving their ordeal, weren't going to end up at a calf ranch or in a veal crate—that was clear. A local family adopted one of the calves, and the three others came to our Orland shelter.

When the calves, whom we named Murray, Mack, and Miles, arrived after their long drive they were moved to a "hospital" pen to be checked for diseases and to get acclimated to their new surroundings. Almost as soon as they arrived, Murray, Mack, and Miles aroused great interest in our resident herd. Many of the adult cattle, both female and male, came down from their barn, craned their necks over the fence, and mooed their welcomes. Murray, Mack, and Miles were quickly learning how to be cattle, so they mooed right back.

Initially, the shelter staff bottle-fed the calves until they were weaned and began to eat grain, hay, and alfalfa. After seven months at the sanctuary, the three were healthy enough to be adopted out to Terri Crisp and her family, near Sacramento. Terri had a number of rescued companion animals along with two young daughters eager to take care of the new arrivals. Murray, Mack, and Miles are there today, on a property with trees and hills and lots of lush grass, and no blue Chevy Impalas in sight. The driver of the Impala told authorities that he had been given the calves by a friend, an Arizona dairy farmer, and didn't see a problem with how he was transporting them. He was charged with a felony but pleaded guilty to lesser charges and was sentenced to six days in jail, one for each of the calves he had stuffed into the trunk of his car. Such is the value of calves under our current laws.

Terri provides regular updates on how Murray, Mack, and Miles are doing. In one she wrote: "I work out of my home and the boys often spend their afternoons lying in the sun outside my office, hoping I won't forget treat time. . . . These three contented cows love the companionship of people and other animals. Our miniature dachshund, Brinkley, seems to be their favorite. I catch them occasionally standing nose to nose with this dog, who is a fraction of their size, as if they were sharing some important secret." I recently had the opportunity to visit the Arizona Humane Society's shelter in Phoenix and was impressed with the facility. Not only had they constructed a barn to provide shelter for various animals, including farm animals, but they also displayed literature about eating vegetarian foods. The Arizona Humane Society is concerned about animals other than just cats and dogs, and this is indicative of a growing awareness within the humane community about the importance of protecting farm animals from abuse.

Of course, the saga of Murray, Mack, and Miles is just one of many cruelty cases involving calves that Farm Sanctuary has come across over the years. Happy endings like these are rare, as is someone, in this case the car's driver, receiving even minimal punishment for the offense.

For male calves in the United States, the future is unclear. The beef industry's use of Holstein calves has provided dairy operators with more potential takers for its "surplus" calves. As a result, the cost of male calves has risen in recent years. This, in turn, has led to increased pressure on the veal industry's bottom line. In the end, competition for baby male calves and consumer disgust may well drive the "milk-fed" veal industry out of business. While it's far from ideal for the calves to end up as beef cattle, what I have seen of the milk-fed veal industry makes even calf ranching look better. If crated, anemic veal production dies out, I, for one, won't miss it at all.

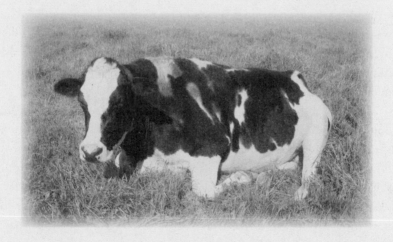

Henry

PROFILE: HENRY

In 1994, I rescued a frail baby calf, a Holstein with a white face framed by black spots, from a crate at a calf ranch. He was only a few days old and had been born on a dairy farm. I was in southern

California, near my parents' home in L.A., which became a temporary refuge for the calf. Actress Kim Basinger had agreed to film a public service announcement (PSA) on downed animals for Farm Sanctuary that would costar this rescued calf. "He should be with his mother" was the first thing Kim, a mother herself, said when I told her about him. "You're right," I replied, thinking that her instinct was exactly on point, "but the dairies take the calves away from their mothers." I went on to explain more about the practices of the dairy industry and calf ranches.

When Kim arrived at my parents' house for the filming, the calf was in the backyard. A longtime advocate for animals, Kim took to him, and he to her, immediately. There were probably a dozen people standing around, but Kim walked right over to the calf. She lay down in the grass with him and began stroking him. Then she asked if he had a name. Not yet, I told her, and I offered to let her do the honors. She had just been reading the work of Henry David Thoreau and decided the calf should be Henry. That PSA begins with Kim asking, "Do you know that animals too sick to walk are still used for human food?"

When she said the line in the script that read "Every living thing feels pain and should be protected from cruelty—farm animals are no different," Henry would moo. Kim read that line a couple times as we did the takes, and each time Henry mooed, right on cue. The camera was rolling and we could see Kim suppressing the urge to laugh—it was as if Henry felt something when he heard her repeat that line. I don't know quite what was going on that afternoon, but I believe in intuition and that we have ways of communicating with animals that go beyond language. Perhaps Henry sensed that Kim really felt the sentiment in the script, and he responded to that.

With the PSA completed, Kim generously became Henry's sponsor, and she sends a check each year to help cover the costs of his care. In the meantime, Henry, a happy resident of the Orland shelter, now weighs in at over two thousand pounds. He gets plenty of fresh air and grass to graze on, and he has many friends within the herd. And yes, he is always ready for his close-up.

CHAPTER EIGHT

How Now Milk Cow?

Hardly any male calves in the United States today live lives like those of Murray, Mack, and Miles. Oddly enough, it was because of the cruelty they had suffered that they escaped confinement and then slaughter. Their mothers, left behind on industrial dairy farms, surely don't get that kind of a break.

Since the wholesale industrialization of farming began after the end of World War II, dairy cows have been bred into and treated like milk machines. According to USDA statistics, in 1950 the average U.S. dairy cow produced 5,700 pounds of milk a year. That's nearly 16 pounds a day, equal to the weight of a good-sized bowling ball. Twenty-five years later, the average had almost doubled, to 10,360 pounds. By 1992, as we were investigating the California dairies in earnest, it had risen to 15,423 pounds. By 2005, in the twenty-three main milk-producing states, more than eight million cows were each pumping out 19,857 pounds of milk a year. That's an extraordinary average of 53 pounds of milk per cow every day, and more than three times as much milk as dairy cows were producing half a century ago.

While some milk carton labels show cows or calves gamboling in green pastures, a growing number of U.S. dairy cows now live in paddocks without pasture, or in stalls inside large sheds that may or may not be open to the outdoors. Rarely, if ever, do they munch on fresh grass. If you know where to look, you can see these factory dairies in traditional milk-producing states such as California, New York, and Wisconsin. They've also moved into places such as New Mexico, which now boasts the largest average dairy farm size in the country. Use your nose, and you'll know when you're coming close to one: the stench of all that manure is impossible to ignore. People living near intensive dairies have called that odor the smell of money.

So many cows producing so much manure in such concentrated conditions means waste disposal is a significant challenge. The sixteen hundred dairies in California's Central Valley alone produce more waste than a city of twenty-one million people—that's more than the populations of London, New York, and Chicago combined. Each cow produces 120 pounds of wet manure per day. In addition, these huge operations are prone to outbreaks of disease and infestation. Drugs and medications, along with harsh antimicrobial chemicals, are routinely used.

All that manure—and the smell that comes with it—is understandably something most people would rather not have move in next door. That's one reason these facilities are continuously being relocated. It's also why many states have enacted what are known as right-to-farm laws that protect agricultural enterprises from liability, despite the harm they can cause to neighbors and communities. At both dairy and beef feedlots in the Southwest, if you can see the pens, you'll see manure, too. Sometimes it's pushed into a mound in the middle of the animals' paddock. During the rainless summer months it dries up and can become airborne in the breeze. At facilities that use liquid manure systems, operators build huge lagoons (a more accurate term would be *cesspools*), which are filled with the cows' waste and the water used to flush that waste from the barn. The quantity of waste produced by all those cows is so large that it's nearly impossible to dispose of it all responsibly—and some people just can't resist a shortcut. On a trip to southern California during the rainy season, I talked to a guy who worked at a dairy farm about their waste management practices. "When the federal boys go home," he told me matter-of-factly, "we just open these spigots and pour this out on the streets."

Of course, the effects aren't so easily washed away. In southern California, where many of these mega-dairies have been located, the groundwater has been polluted by waste and wastewater. Agricultural producers have preferential access to water, so when they sell their land along with the water rights to developers, they get a premium price for it, even if the groundwater is contaminated. Water is a valuable commodity in the arid West and Southwest, and residential and commercial developers are so eager to obtain water rights that they're willing to pay to clean up the dairies' pollution. The result is that dairy farmers buy land for their operations, pollute the water, and then sell when the property value goes up. They use the profits to purchase land in less populated areas where there are fewer neighbors to complain about the manure. Then the cycle starts all over again. Because California's population is projected to grow by more than twelve million people—to more than forty-six million— by 2030, demand for suburban housing is only going to increase and expand the life of this cycle.

The sheer size of the dairies can lead to other problems. During the heat wave that hit California in July 2006, more than a hundred people died, along with about 25,000 dairy cows (as well as 700,000 chickens and 160,000 turkeys). So many cows' bodies were piling up that six counties declared states of emergency, and the Department of Food and Agriculture waived its regulation that the dead cows be transported to rendering plants in the Central Valley. Instead, the department authorized farmers to dump cows' bodies in local landfills. "If you don't bury them, you have to deal with the stench and flies," John Ferreira of the Cotta & Ferreira Dairy in Stockton told the *San Francisco Chronicle*. The industry also noted that the cows weren't giving their usual high yields. "Cows don't want to eat as much when it's hot," Ferreira added. "[B]ut if they are not eating, they are not producing milk. It goes hand in hand."

The Secret Lives of Dairy Cows

Dairy cows, like other mammals, produce milk after giving birth. They are kept pregnant virtually all the time and usually give birth to a calf each year. Like humans, a cow's gestation period is nine months. For seven of those months, she is also producing milk. But because she simply wouldn't be able to deliver the amount of milk the industry expects while also providing nutrients to her growing fetus, she is fed a meal of high-energy concentrates. That's not all she eats. For years, dairy and beef cows were fed meat and bone meal from dead cows, until scientists established that the practice could spread mad cow disease. While some restrictions have been put in place in recent years, the cows can still be fed manure from poultry operations, along with fish meal, feather meal, and urea, an organic compound derived from mammals' urine. You would think that even factory farmers would balk at feeding this revolting mix of blood, guts, and manure to herbivores, but apparently they don't.

This strange diet and the demands on their bodies mean that industrialized dairy cows regularly suffer from a number of diseases. One is milk fever (or hypocalcemia), which results from inadequate calcium in the cow's blood. The excretion of milk drains the cow's calcium stores faster than the cow can replenish them, and she falls ill, sometimes fatally so. Milk fever tends to afflict cows right after they've given birth. Another common result of their high-energy feed is ketosis, which causes the cow to lose weight, produce less milk, and become infertile—all of which are the equivalent of a death sentence for a cow in today's dairy industry.

Other means the dairy industry uses to boost milk production carry risks for the cows and for us. In 1993, for example, the U.S. Food and Drug Administration (FDA) approved the use of the synthetic version of a naturally occurring hormone called recombinant bovine growth hormone (or rBGH). rBGH was developed to increase milk yields in dairy cows, and it worked remarkably well, raising milk volume by as much as 40 percent. Although rBGH is banned in Canada, Australia, New Zealand, and some European countries, according to the manufacturer Monsanto, one-third of all dairy cattle in all fifty U.S. states have been injected with the hormone, which it sells under the name Posilac. Since the mid-1990s, consumer advocates concerned about its effects on human health have demanded that the U.S. government mandate that milk products with rBGH be labeled. Given the widespread use of hormones and antibiotics in the meat industries, these activists have good reason to be up in arms. But the government has refused these requests for accurate labeling, insisting there is no evidence that rBGH entering the milk supply causes problems for people.

While public health and consumer advocates continue to debate what rBGH does, or may do, to the human body, there's no doubt that it causes problems for cows. According to Canadian researchers, the use of rBGH has increased rates of mastitis by 40 percent. Mastitis is an extremely painful udder infection that is potentially fatal in advanced stages. At the same time, the incidence of infertility has gone up by nearly 20 percent. In addition, rBGH increased by 50 percent cases of laminitis, a hoof ailment that is intensely painful and makes it hard for cows to stand. In order to treat mastitis and other negative consequences of rBGH, farmers are forced to use even more medications and antibiotics. (Cows are given antibiotics not only to prevent or treat disease but also routinely as an agent to improve feed conversion efficiency; in other words, with antibiotics, cows produce more milk on less feed.)

Consumers' concerns about drinking milk with added hormones such as rBGH and their frustration at being kept in the dark have helped create a flourishing organic milk and dairy products industry. While only 3.5 percent of dairy products sold in the United States are organic, both the food industry and consumer associations expect that to grow. Indeed, in 2005 its value was put at $2.1 billion by the Organic Trade Association, up 24 percent from the year before.

One positive outcome of this demand is that some organic dairy farmers have gone back to basics. Their cows aren't penned but instead graze on pasture. They eat organic feed, free of antibiotics, and they receive no hormone injections. These organic dairies are small in scale and more like the family farms of old. In some cases, the cows are given names by the farmer and his or her family. This is a welcome development and a departure from the attitude of a California dairyman who told *The New York Times,* "On a lot of those farms in the Midwest and back east, every cow has a name. . . . It's not like that here. A cow's a piece of machinery. If it's broke, we try to fix it, and if it can't, it gets replaced."

Unfortunately, the story of organic farming has a downside. A new beast is emerging: the corporate-style organic dairy farm. Cows at those operations aren't given hormones or antibiotics, but their feed is mostly grain and, as in a feedlot or factory farm, the animals don't have access to pasture or much space to graze. Some of these farms have more than four thousand cows. The same economic forces at play in conventional agriculture that have led industrialized production to undermine family farms are threatening organic agriculture. It's especially sad to see this happening in the organics industry, which originally seemed to offer a better way. On the other hand, advocates—for consumers, for organics, for family farms, and for farmed animals—are speaking out and voting with their dollars. The Organic Consumers Association has launched a boycott against Horizon, the largest organic milk brand in the United States, to protest its purchase of milk from "organic" cows raised in feedlot conditions. (Aurora Organic Dairy, which supplies organic milk to large chains such as Costco and Safeway, has also met with criticism for raising dairy cows in feedlot-like facilities.) The USDA is working on standards for organic dairy products; one draft version would require that the cows spend at least 120 days during the year on pasture. However, large-scale "organic" dairies are actively lobbying to weaken the standards.

Given the enormous strain put on dairy cows' bodies and the various maladies that come from intensive production, it's not surprising that most no longer live the fifteen or twenty years they did in pre-factory-farming days (and that the cows at Farm Sanctuary do). Today, most dairy cows are in production for only a few years before they are trucked off to slaughter. Many are so sick they can't stand, and so they become downers. Their bodies are so spent that dairy cows aren't considered a source of high-quality meat. Most of them become hamburger.

The large number of downed dairy cows has not escaped the notice of some dairy industry insiders. One of them is Dr. Jim Reynolds, who, you'll remember, supported the California downed animal bill. Dr. Reynolds saw what was happening to downed dairy cows as an affront to his profession as a veterinarian and his conscience. Jim also supported other efforts to prevent the suffering of downed cows and legislation to stop the intensive confinement of calves raised for milk-fed veal production. Like a growing number of individuals in the industry, Jim corroborated what I had seen, and he felt these practices were simply wrong and had to be stopped. One day, Jim made a pained request that I could tell came from his heart: "Please make this go away."

Unfortunately, for his courageous and compassionate stance Dr. Reynolds was ostracized by members of his industry, particularly the Farm Bureau, which contacted his dairy farm clients and urged them to fire Jim. The criticism reached such a pitch that it damaged Jim's relationship with some of his dairies. He now works as a dairy clinician with the Veterinary Teaching and Research Center at the University of California, Davis. Compassion like Jim's is, unfortunately, still too short in supply, even among veterinarians. Too few in his vocation have the courage to stand up to industry and be true to their professional oath.

During the California no-downer campaign, I was talking to the manager of a slaughterhouse, this time wearing (figuratively speaking) my Cornell agricultural economics graduate hat. "As these animal people continue talking about this downed animal thing," I said, "don't you think it might make sense for you to stop accepting downed animals? It gives you guys a black eye," I continued. "Makes you look irresponsible, and it's something that is upsetting the consumers."

The manager shrugged. "Well, let's put it this way," he said. "If your wife was sick and you'd get $500 by bringing her here, would you do that or would you kill her at home?"

My jaw dropped. How do you reply to a question like that? What I'm sure the manager meant to say, or I hope he meant to say, was this: that the animals were worth money and that it made sense to transport them to a slaughterhouse where he could at least walk away with a few more dollars in his wallet—no matter how sick they were—rather than be euthanized on the farm. No financial return in that scenario. Given the emphasis on production, production, production that affects every corner of agribusiness, I'll never be sure whether the slaughterhouse manager really thought that was an apt analogy. If every aspect of your life is governed by the bottom line, then all life, no matter whose it is or what condition it's in, can be a source of profit, a commodity for sale. Accepting institutionalized animal cruelty as a cost of doing business requires a flexible conscience, and I guess we shouldn't be surprised when the same attitude starts slipping into the way we think about each other.

In the Name of Commerce

We tend to think of cows as gentle, passive creatures, and for the most part they are. Cattle like to ruminate and chew their cud—it's part of their way of digesting—and it's no accident that when we're feeling in a reflective mood we say we're "ruminating" or "chewing on a thought." On the other hand, beef cattle have retained more of their wild spirit.

Despite the practices and preferences of the industry, cows are still cows and share fundamental natures and many similarities in behavior (when these behaviors can be expressed). At both of our shelters, we have beef and dairy cattle and they get along fine within the herds. What we've found is that beef and dairy cows can be placid as well as strong and independent, particularly when they want to get out of an unpleasant situation they've found themselves in. While some people may consider farmed animals passive and even complicit in accepting the harsh realities of factory farms, we still find ourselves rooting for them when they manage to even temporarily break free.

What we've done to the animals in the name of farming has muddied our view of them as individuals. But no matter how heavily bred or battered, each has his or her own individual personality and, if he or she is allowed to express it, a unique spirit. We may not understand it, but if we pay attention, we can see it.

Three of the cows currently at the Watkins Glen shelter, all of whom were bred for beef, took destiny into their own hands. Cinci Freedom escaped from a slaughterhouse in Cincinnati in 2002; Queenie broke out of a halal slaughterhouse in Queens, New York, in 2000; and Annie Dodge spent weeks on the run in 2005 after escaping from a stockyard in Vermont before she ended up in the yard of two Farm Sanctuary supporters. You may even remember hearing about them. All had their day in the media spotlight and were saved by an outpouring of public sympathy.

Although beef cattle such as these slaughterhouse escapees are also factory farmed, they tend to lead the least constrained lives of all farmed animals. I don't mean to say the thirty million cattle slaughtered each year for beef in the United States are living the life of Riley. Cow-calf operators at the beginning of the beef production chain keep cows on the range, and may have one bull for many cows. The cows will be naturally bred, and the calves will nurse from their mothers for perhaps six months before they are taken away, an event no less stressful for a mother and child at 180 days than it is a day after birth. Temple Grandin has described how, when calves are taken from their mothers, mother and calf alike will sometimes "bellow themselves hoarse."

The male calves are castrated—without painkillers—and these steers are then raised for beef. Both male and female calves are generally "disbudded," which means their "bud," the beginning of their horn, is removed, also without painkillers. Beef producers are now breeding cattle

without horns (called polled breeds) to eliminate the need for this procedure. Female calves are either raised for beef or, if they're thought to be
good breeders, kept on the pasture to expand the herd. If she fails to breed
and produce calves, or if she is simply too old, a female cow will be sent to
slaughter and replaced with a younger cow for the breeding herd.

Cattle today don't spend their lives eating grass on the prairie as they
once did. Even if they are born on the range, they are moved to feedlots,
where most beef cattle spend the last six months of their lives. On feedlots, thousands of cows are crowded into manure-laden holding pens
where they stand on the trampled earth. There's no pasture or any trees
to provide shade, and because the air is thick with harmful bacteria and
particulate matter, the cattle are at constant risk of contracting respiratory diseases. They are fed grain concentrates to encourage rapid, unnatural weight gain—in fact, the average cow will consume more than
three thousand pounds of grain during his or her stay. The feedlots are
so packed that, as Eric Schlosser describes in his book *Fast Food Nation*,
they look like "a sea of cattle, a mooing, moving mass of brown and
white fur that goes on for acres."

Because cattle are biologically suited to eat a grass-based, high-fiber
diet, their concentrated feedlot rations contribute to metabolic disorders
and other ailments. Sick and diseased livestock are a common sight on
feedlots, and veterinary care is generally inadequate or nonexistent. In
the 1950s, farmers began using growth hormones to increase weight gain
in their cattle. Today, more than 90 percent of U.S. cattle on feedlots are
implanted with hormones. Cattle on the range do have pasture to graze
on, but their living conditions aren't ideal. They aren't protected against
inclement weather and may die of dehydration or freeze to death; often,
they give birth on frozen or snowy ground. In addition, injured, ill, or
otherwise ailing cattle rarely receive necessary veterinary attention on
the range.

Whether fattened in feedlots or on the range, when they are trucked
to slaughter or to stockyards or auctions many cattle experience stress
and injury. Some will become downers. Cattle may be transported several times during their lifetimes, and they may be hauled hundreds or even
thousands of miles on a single trip, without food or water. It is both legal
and common for animals to remain on transport trucks for twenty-eight

hours or even more. Every year, many thousands of cattle and calves die in transit in the United States.

There's a final indignity at the slaughterhouse. Modern beef slaughterhouses kill up to four hundred head of cattle every hour. The high speed of the assembly line makes it increasingly difficult to provide animals with any semblance of humane treatment before and as they die. In April 2001, a *Washington Post* article described the conditions at a cattle slaughter plant in gruesome detail:

> The cattle were supposed to be dead before they got to Moreno [a slaughterhouse worker]. But too often they weren't.
>
> They blink. They make noises, he said softly. The head moves, the eyes are wide and looking around. Still Moreno would cut. On bad days, he says, dozens of animals reached his station clearly alive and conscious. Some would survive as far as the tail cutter, the belly ripper, the hide puller. They die, said Moreno, piece by piece.

You've already read about how veal calves are taken from their mothers (dairy cows) almost as soon as they are born. For beef cows, the experience of losing their calves is no less wrenching. Even though the industry claims that the mothering instinct has been bred out of the cows, my experiences tell me otherwise. I've documented cows being separated from their calves, and if they're not resisting, then I don't know what it is. Separating the pairs often requires prodding, pushing, yelling, and eventually restraints. I've heard many farmers talk about an ornery or angry cow butting and kicking handlers to try to keep her calf at her side. I remember seeing a downed cow at a Texas stockyard whose neck had been injured in the struggle to keep her calf. Her head was crooked back and rested limply on one shoulder. She was shaking in pain and fear. It upsets me just thinking of it.

I have seen the way the cows at Farm Sanctuary care for young calves and form lifelong bonds. It doesn't matter whether they've given birth or haven't, whether they are beef or dairy breeds; they still care for the young. I've even seen cows become surrogate mothers to members of other species. Phoebe is a case in point. In 1997, she was rescued with twenty-one other cows from a rundown dairy farm where she and the others had been kept in a dirty warehouse, starved, and not properly milked or provided with veterinary care.

When Phoebe came to Farm Sanctuary we saw that she had a chronic leg problem. As a special-needs cow, she lived in the sheep barn with other special-needs cows, who weren't strong enough to butt heads or keep up with the scampering of other members of the herd. Sheep are smaller and gentler than cattle, so they make good companions for these cows.

Phoebe became fast friends with a sheep named David who was sixteen years old when he was rescued. Sixteen is ancient for a sheep, and David was sick. Phoebe obviously decided that David needed special care, too, and she became his constant companion. She would lick him and gently try to herd him. She became so protective that she would try to butt the shelter staff when they came to give David his medication. At sixteen hundred pounds, Phoebe was a formidable foe, and our caregivers had to separate them each day for a short time while David got the treatments he needed. Even then, Phoebe didn't leave David. She would reach her head through the stall gate and lick him the whole time. One day, the staff took too long for Phoebe's tastes. She busted two gate latches trying to get to her sheep friend. If David wandered too far out of Phoebe's sight when they were grazing in the pastures together, Phoebe would cry out loudly, and David would return to her. At night, the two bedded down together in thick straw, lying side by side as they slept.

David's illness, however, got worse, and one night he died. Phoebe just wouldn't accept it. When the staff arrived in the morning, they found Phoebe nuzzling David, trying over and over again to get him to stand up. We couldn't wait long before we had to bury him, and we hoped that somehow Phoebe would recognize that David was dead and be all right.

But Phoebe wasn't okay. In fact, she spent the next twelve hours walking up and down, mooing at the other sheep as if asking for David. I think anyone who believes cows don't have feelings should hear the sound of a cow in grief: it is an unearthly wail that is impossible to ignore. In fact, in Phoebe's case it was so heart-wrenching that we brought David's body back into the barn. It relieved her, but no matter how much she nudged him, David wasn't going to get up. Finally, we took David away and buried him.

For a week, Phoebe looked for him. During that time, she refused to eat. We were so concerned that she would starve to death that we locked her in a pen with food and water. While she did eventually begin to eat and drink again, Phoebe never truly recovered from David's death. You could see she had simply lost the will to live. After a year, Phoebe was still sick with grief, and her leg condition had worsened to the point that she could no longer stand. We made the difficult decision to euthanize her. We felt that at some level that was what she wanted.

We'll never know how many calves had been taken away from Phoebe before she came to Farm Sanctuary or how often she had had to mourn this loss. Perhaps David's death was just one blow too many. When farmers or scientists assert that animals don't feel loss or can't express love, or suggest that they are indifferent to life or death, I think of Phoebe and David. When you watch animals go through that kind of pain, when you hear them bellowing and lowing at the loss of a companion or a baby, you know that it is both bad science and bad farming to turn a blind eye to their experience of loss. When you see the fear or panic that I have seen in the eyes of cows and other animals as they are penned in stockyards or on their way to slaughter, you can see how much they want to live and be free. In this regard, they are not very different from cats and dogs and other companion animals—and us.

The animals at the shelters in Orland and Watkins Glen express the full spectrum of emotions and character traits. They are as playful, curmudgeonly, devious, kindhearted, intelligent, lazy, and aggressive as some of us. In a very elemental way, they're not that different from us after all, except in one particular: they seem to embody a purity in being alive that many of us, sadly, seem to have lost.

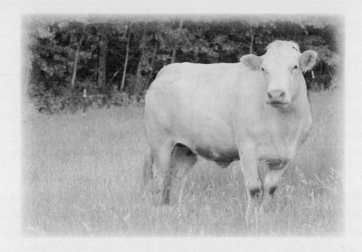

Cinci Freedom

PROFILE: CINCI FREEDOM

In the late winter of 2002, Cinci Freedom, a spirited white Charolais cow, ran for her life—literally. Little did she know when she leaped a six-foot fence at an Ohio slaughterhouse that she'd become a national cause célèbre. Raised as a beef cow, Cinci (short for Cincinnati) was relatively small and lean, and she could jump. That particular jump got her out of the slaughter line and into a nearly two-week sojourn in Cincinnati's wooded Mount Storm Park, during which time she eluded repeated attempts to capture her and also, as a reporter for *The Cincinnati Enquirer* wrote, "reminded Cincinnatians where pot roast comes from."

Cinci's freedom run so captivated the city, and indeed the country, that this cow destined for the dinner table was given a reprieve. The meat company to which Cinci belonged agreed to surrender its rights to her, and thanks to the generosity of iconic artist Peter Max, a vegan and environmentalist, Cinci Freedom came to live at Farm Sanctuary's Watkins Glen shelter. Before she came to us, Cinci received the key to the city after which she's named from then-mayor Charlie Luken—the

first cow to be honored in this way that I know of. Peter later presented his portrait of Cinci to the city, and it was hung in City Hall. He also
pledged to raise funds through his artwork for the local SPCA.

Since her arrival, Cinci's wounds have healed and she's put on some
weight. But she hasn't lost any of her spirit or her agility. Cinci's not
a large cow, just over a thousand pounds, but she's tough when she
needs to be. She has become friendly with several of the females in the
farm's main herd, including another slaughterhouse escapee and cow
celebrity, Queenie, from New York City. Cinci is, though, still wary of
people. She carefully watches everything the caretakers are doing—she
doesn't miss a beat—and they know to stay far enough away from her
so she won't feel threatened. Cinci can still jump; she's easily cleared the
pasture fences when she's wanted to avoid the visiting hoof trimmer.

Our farming neighbors warned us that Cinci was dangerous and
would surely hurt someone. As far as they were concerned, we never
should have taken her in. What really gets to Cinci, we've found, is being cornered. Since she was in a slaughterhouse line when she jumped
to freedom, that's not surprising. We've found ways to get her the care
she needs without putting her into a pen. I admire Cinci's tenacity and
her resilience. She's made sure she'll not be pushed around by anyone
or anything ever again.

CHAPTER NINE

It's Not
Wilbur's Farm Anymore

The swine unit manager at the University of Florida in Gainesville said something else the day I met him that has stayed with me. As I was leaving his office, he turned to me and declared in a clear, even tone, "You know what everybody should see? A sow build a nest."

I was surprised to hear him say it—and couldn't agree with him more. At Farm Sanctuary, sows build nests every day, taking fresh straw in their mouths and moving it into a pile. In the winter, they burrow under the straw and sleep. When it's hot they gather less straw and lie on top instead of under it. At the end of a long day, I love to unwind in the pig barn, listening to the pigs' rhythmic breathing and contented snoring.

In a natural setting, sows' nests are bedded with grasses, leaves, and other materials from the surrounding environment. The sow gathers and carries this to a sheltered location, where she gives birth. She keeps her piglets in the nest until they are on their feet, and then introduces them to other sows and their offspring. Pigs raise their young cooperatively in groups, taking turns watching over the piglets. When danger approaches, they band together to protect their young.

Unlike grazing animals, such as herd-oriented sheep and cattle, pigs are more individualistic. In my experience, they're more like human beings than any other farm animal. They develop one-on-one relationships, and even social cliques, that last for years. They favor certain pig peers over others. Pigs have extremely sensitive noses and a highly attuned sense of smell. They love to root around in the soil and dig their hooves and bodies into the earth. They create wallows in wet areas for mud baths. Because they don't have sweat glands, they use the mud to cool off.

Winston Churchill knew what he was talking about when he once said, "I like pigs. Dogs look up to us. Cats look down on us. Pigs treat us as equals." Contrary to common lore about pigs, their homes are not "sties." Pigs are, in fact, very clean. At the Farm Sanctuary shelters, almost all of the pigs use the center of their barns as a communal toilet rather than the straw where they sleep. It's relatively easy to clean up after them.

Pigs are actually very regimented creatures: certain pigs eat first, and each sleeps in a specific location. Pig hierarchies are not based on physical strength alone. Boots, for instance, is the oldest pig at the shelter in Watkins Glen. She has been weakened by age and couldn't defend herself if other pigs wanted to push her around. But none of the other pigs ever tries. All of them treat their wise elder with respect.

Like people, pigs can develop rivalries, and sometimes we need to separate them. When we can, we adopt out those who are not getting along with the rest of the herd. We adopt animals—including pigs—out in groups of no less than two to ensure they'll be with a companion of their species.

Pigs are among the most vocal farm animals and can make a lot of noise: they scream when they're afraid or angry, and will grunt their contentment when you rub their bellies or stroke their ears. Their eyes are very much like ours. When you look into a pig's eyes, you can see their emotions, maybe even their souls. The eyes show fear and vulnerability, and also joy and satisfaction.

Pigs can be very loyal—as well as ornery. When Farm Sanctuary's home was the tofu farm in Pennsylvania, we rescued a number of pigs, including Hope. She had been abandoned in the loading dock at Lancaster Stockyards with a badly broken leg. Hope had a sweet disposition and watched patiently as we put food in front of her before digging in and grunting appreciatively. Unfortunately, because of Hope's lame leg, some of our other pigs, especially the slightly greedy Raquel, would generally get to the food first. (It sort of reminded me of being at the dinner table with my five brothers and sisters.) If I happened to be on hand, I could keep Raquel from stealing Hope's food. But without supervision, it was another story. Several times I fed the pigs and then made as if to leave the barn but secretly stood observing them from a distance. Raquel would stand with her ears, eyes, and nose alert, trying to work out whether I'd actually left so that she could get away with feasting on Hope's food. It was clear she knew she was doing something she wasn't supposed to, and wanted to make sure she didn't get caught.

While other pigs came to Hope's aid, we kept an eye on her until the arrival of Johnny. A younger and newly rescued pig, he quickly became Hope's loyal companion and protector. At feeding time, Johnny stayed by Hope's side to make sure she ate without any interference. At night, the pair slept side by side. Hope was much older than Johnny, and as the years went by, Hope's health deteriorated and she eventually died. Johnny was despondent. Though still young and healthy, he died a couple of weeks later. The only explanation I can come up with is that he died of a broken heart.

Inside an Industrial Pork Farm

While I can't say for sure that pigs in industrial farms die of broken hearts, I can tell you that they die of heart attacks. And I can also tell you what these facilities look like. They're a far cry from the roomy barns and pasture at Farm Sanctuary. In a factory pig operation, every decision is guided by efficiency of production. Imagine a long, low, windowless shed. If it's a shed for breeding sows, inside you'd see a warehouse-like space filled by row after row of two-foot-wide metal crates. In the distance, all you see are bars and tubes and machinery. The animals have disappeared from sight into what writer Matthew Scully calls "a sunless hell of metal and concrete."

You would, however, smell the pigs as well as hear them. An overwhelming stench of ammonia and a cacophony of shrieks and squeals are common. You'll also hear fans, which turn on automatically when the temperature hits a certain threshold. If you were to step up, you'd see in each crate a sow, along with a trough for food and a metal nipple (for water) at the front. Beneath the pigs are slatted concrete floors; the pig manure falls through the slats into pits below, which are then flushed into nearby lagoons. The toxic brew may later be sprayed onto adjacent fields or become a fertile breeding ground for insects. Not long ago, through the skills of a forensic entomologist, a community demonstrated that their homes had been infested with drone flies (adult rattail maggots) from nearby hog manure lagoons. They won a judgment of $5 million.

In front and behind each row of sows are alleyways just wide enough for workers to pass through. In addition to monitoring feed and water at the front, the workers hose down manure at the back. Even then, manure piles up and becomes caked to the concrete slats of the floor in between cleanings. The pigs can't escape lying in it.

On industrial farms, the pigs are injected with minerals (such as iron) and given antibiotics to encourage faster growth. If allowed outdoors, pigs would obtain essential nutrients, including iron, from the soil. Clipped on the front of the crates are sheets that identify the sow and list when she was bred, her treatment and production schedule, and her due date. Each sow is merely a production unit. This is the reality of the sows' lives, day after day, week after week. It's no surprise that physical and psychological problems are common.

I've had the misfortune of visiting pig factories across the United States and have seen thousands of confined sows. Pigs are curious by nature and easily bored. There is literally nothing for them to do in these facilities. The sows can't walk, turn around, or lie down comfortably. I've seen some motionless, depressed, and unresponsive to anything around them. They appeared to be suffering from a learned helplessness, similar to what people can experience when they lose hope and give up trying to escape a bad situation because every attempt they've made to help themselves has been fruitless. In other cases, I've seen confined sows stressed out and agitated. They gnaw at the metal bars of their crates, press their snouts against the front of their enclosures, or move their heads from side to side. For years, animal welfare scientists have discussed this "repetitive, useless behavior" as a neurotic coping mechanism animals show in response to "confined, isolated (for social animals), or deprived environments."

In defending gestation crates, the pork industry is quick to argue that the alternatives are worse. They say, for example, that when

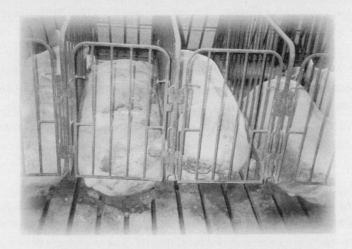

Pigs' gestation crates

sows are kept in group housing systems they become aggressive toward each other. However, farmers who take account of the animals' social system and honor the relationships between them are able to manage group housing systems with few problems. I've visited pig farms where sows are kept in groups, and haven't seen fights or signs of them (such as bite marks). However, a group housing system cannot be used halfheartedly or ignorantly. What is required is a greater understanding of the animals, that is, pigmanship.

The sows do get to leave the gestation crates—but only to be crammed into another. Near the end of her four-month pregnancy, a sow is moved into what is called a "farrowing crate" to give birth and (briefly) nurse her young. The farrowing crates are similar to the gestation crates: the floors are typically hard metal grating, with holes to allow waste to fall through. The mother stands or lies on her side while her piglets nurse from under the metal bars. Pork industry public relations people claim that these farrowing crates prevent sows from lying on and smothering their piglets. But the problem may be the crates themselves. Unable to move freely or turn around, crated sows have a limited awareness of their immediate environment, including where their piglets are. As a result, they typically lie down awkwardly (read: fast and hard), and their piglets, who weigh just a few pounds at birth, can be easily injured or killed if they happen to be in the wrong place at the wrong time.

Mortality rates for piglets in these systems are high. Approximately 15 percent die. Roughly half of these deaths are attributed to crushing by the sow. That's not the only danger piglets face. They sometimes literally fall through the cracks in the crate floors into the waste system below. I have heard that officials in Ithaca, New York, have complained to Cornell University on more than one occasion because piglets from the university's swine unit were flushed into the city's sewage system and their bodies clogged up the pipes.

On commercial farms, a piglet's life follows a prescribed pattern. They are removed from their mothers anywhere between one and four weeks after birth to be fattened for slaughter. The sooner the piglets can be weaned, the sooner the sow can be reimpregnated. These events are timed to fit the production schedule and to stimulate the sow's next estrus or "heat." When the time is right she'll be artificially inseminated and spend her new pregnancy, like the last one, in a gestation crate. The semen used to impregnate her is obtained by manually masturbating the boars used for breeding. In her book *Animals in Translation,* Temple Grandin describes what various boars seemed to need to become aroused, including having their backs scratched and other actions that were, as Grandin writes, "a lot more intimate." Outside the world of factory farming, such conduct would be considered depraved and illegal. Inside the world of factory farming, it is normal.

After they are weaned, piglets are raised in nurseries, where the temperature is kept high to keep their still-frail bodies warm. This way feed calories most efficiently fuel growth. Here, at least, the piglets get to live with other piglets. But the pens are crowded, the floors are hard and unnatural, and the piglets have nothing to stimulate them apart from each other. At about two months, they are moved to what are known as "grower houses," which are large complexes of metal pens with slatted and concrete floors.

Compared with their mothers, piglets raised solely for meat live relatively short lives, just six months—in essence, they die in adolescence, since their slaughter age coincides roughly with sexual maturity.

The male pigs are castrated as piglets—without an anesthetic—to avoid wasted energy, an inefficiency, and the hassle of dealing with unwanted pregnancies. Castrating males also results in less pungent-tasting flesh, removing what the industry calls "boar taint," which producers consider undesirable for American consumers. If young sows being fattened for slaughter become pregnant, feed calories are directed to the pregnancy rather than the industry's priority: the growth of salable muscle.

Sickly or slow-growing piglets in the farrowing or fattening facilities have even shorter lives. In 2003, for example, two employees quit their jobs at Smithfield's Circle Four farm in Utah and related what they had seen there to the *Salt Lake Tribune*. The paper quoted the pair as saying that "if a piglet did not weigh at least five pounds after a week, it got 'knocked,' a euphemism for 'beaten to death.' . . . The most common 'knocking' method was to grab the animal by its hind legs and slam it into a wall or concrete floor."

This is "humane euthanasia," factory farm style, and a common practice on pig farms today. The workers made other allegations that make for difficult reading, including fellow employees "beating uncooperative sows with metal rods and improperly castrating newborn pigs." They also said they were disturbed by the assembly-line efficiency of the operation that gave animals little freedom or space to move around.

It's no wonder agribusiness is pushing state legislatures to pass laws making it illegal to enter industrial animal facilities, let alone videotape what goes on. The former Smithfield employees expressed concern about the intensive, prolonged confinement of the sows, and noted that the sows were visibly upset when their piglets were taken away. In spite of their description of the sows' obvious distress, Dr. Paul Sundberg, a veterinarian for the National Pork Board in Washington, D.C., and the same man who'd agreed with me that pigmanship was missing on today's farms, commented, "I'm not sure I would subscribe to the theory that it is a traumatic experience to the mother."

At around three to five years of age, after they have produced four to eight litters, the sows' productivity begins to drop off, and they are shipped to slaughter. In a last assault on these animals' welfare, farmers typically deny the sows feed during their last days, to save a few more cents. Visiting gestation crate facilities and livestock markets over the years, I've seen many "cull sows," their bodies worn out, bruised, and battered from years of confinement.

It's a bad life for pigs, and the workers fare little better. On industrial farms, workers, like animals, are seen as tools of production. When injured or otherwise no longer useful, they're replaced. Just as farmed animals are excluded from laws that protect other animals, farm workers are denied rights that protect other workers—in practice if not by law. And just as a certain percentage of animals are expected to die at various stages of the production cycle, so a certain level of workplace injury is par for the course.

After spending a day at Smithfield's Tar Heel, North Carolina, pork processing plant, where thirty-two thousand hogs are slaughtered daily, *New York Times* columnist Bob Herbert wrote: "[T]he work is brutal beyond imagining. Company officials will tell you everything is fine, but serious injuries abound . . . the processing line on the kill floor moves hogs past the workers at the dizzying rate of one every three or four seconds." The non-unionized workers are nearly all poor and African American, Asian American, or Latino (many are undocumented—no industry is more disdainful of immigration laws). When the United Food and Commercial Workers Union tried to organize workers at the plant, Smithfield, according to a judge, violated federal labor law to stop creation of a union. In 2006 the U.S. Court of Appeals found "intense and widespread coercion prevalent at [Smithfield's] Tar Heel facility" to stifle union activity.

Blaming the Victim

Amazingly, the pigs are blamed for their own confinement. Agricultural scientists and industrial farmers will tell you that sows are uncaring mothers, which is why they step on and harm their own piglets in the farrowing crates. When sows exhibit frustration and become agitated, they are assumed to be violent and dangerous, even if this behavior is the result of their piglets being taken away.

Despite a wealth of evidence to the contrary, I have heard pig farmers explain that it's necessary to confine sows tightly in crates for their own good to prevent them from harming other pigs or people. They also say that the crates promote animal welfare for both piglets and sows. They claim the sows actually *enjoy* the crates and prefer them to being outdoors. Some have gone as far as to suggest that the crates are comfortable and pleasant and have told me they'd trade places with the animals, so luxurious are the accommodations.

Those who take the issue more seriously recognize that much of the scientific evidence cited in defense of using crates compares one bad commercial system to another, and they conclude that neither is good. When I ask animal scientists if they really believe sows would choose to live in gestation crates instead of pastures replete with shade trees and wallowing ponds, they look perplexed. It's as if providing the animals with such conditions had never occurred to them. It doesn't fit the economic model that current agricultural practice considers optimal, so it simply doesn't enter the equation.

In today's price-driven market, the pressure to produce cheap pigs is intense—and concern about animal welfare ranges from minimal to nonexistent. For instance, when veterinarians and other experts were commissioned by the American Veterinary Medical Association (AVMA) to study the welfare of breeding sows, they compared two systems: gestation crates and crowded group housing. They didn't even think about a pasture system. The parameters and mind-set have become frighteningly narrow, with animal welfare concerns brushed aside impatiently by industry-paid veterinarians.

The simple truth is that gestation and farrowing crates are cruel and profoundly unnatural, frustrating the sows' most basic instincts and making healthy mothering impossible. By every measure, they compromise the well-being of both sows and piglets. Standing or lying on concrete and metal grated floors is bad for the pigs' feet, causing painful hoof and leg disorders and lameness, as well as sores on the sows' legs and bodies. Denied the ability to exercise, the sows' muscles atrophy, and this contributes to impaired mobility and bone weakness. Pigs are not given straw or other comfortable bedding because it represents an extra cost and would require additional labor. It also wouldn't fit with the liquid manure systems used on today's hog factories that rely on regular hosing.

In European countries, gestation crates have been outlawed, and they are coming under increasing scrutiny in the United States. Responding to growing public concern, the Food Marketing Institute (FMI) and the National Council of Chain Restaurants (NCCR), which represent the largest retail food outlets in the United States, spoke with industry representatives about developing voluntary guidelines to improve the welfare of pigs and other animals on factory farms. They suggested that gestation crates be at least wide enough to allow the pregnant sow to "be able to lie down on her side without her teats extending into the adjacent stall."

Even such a minimal guideline, however, was apparently too much for some in the pig industry, and it devised a shortcut. In response, the FMI and NCCR issued a statement clarifying that "preventing a sow's teats from extending into another sow's crate should not be achieved by compressing the udder with a wall, bar or other barrier." The FMI-NCCR effort to improve farmed animal welfare seems to have gotten bogged down, and industry groups have begun creating their own, extremely weak, voluntary welfare guidelines.

Pig Tales

Every day at Farm Sanctuary we interact with pigs. To us, they aren't dangerous animals, or bad mothers, or dirty, messy "hogs" with diseases or bad attitudes or insatiable appetites. I'm happy that other people are also beginning to see them in a different light. Visitors to Farm Sanctuary in particular are getting a chance to know the pigs, as well as the other animals at our shelters, for who they really are.

Some years ago, a pig farmer visited us in Watkins Glen. He saw two young women volunteers, each of whom probably weighed about a hundred pounds, cleaning a barn and working around five-hundred-pound sows. "Be careful," he warned the women. "One of those pigs will knock you down and the other will have your guts in a second." He was genuinely alarmed and believed the women were in a dangerous situation.

The farmer described an incident when a sow came after him, "shattering a four-by-four post like it was a toothpick," after he took her piglets away. I urged the man to calm down and explained that our sows didn't attack people and that they actually enjoyed being around us. While some of the animals who come to Farm Sanctuary are initially fearful of human beings, I told him, when they were treated with compassion they learned to trust people and became comfortable in their surroundings. Over the years, I've found this consistently to be the case. When shown kindness, the animals typically respond in kind, despite what they've been through. In this way, they mirror our own behavior.

It's always interesting what people see in the animals. Some of the pigs at our shelters are huge—as long as small couches. They can weigh nine hundred pounds or more and have enormous rear ends. They've been bred to grow to such sizes so that their bodies provide more of the parts people like to eat. A few years ago, a former football player visited. When he went into the pig barn, he stopped short and exclaimed, "These pigs remind me of my football buddies." His friends, he explained, had taken hormones to increase their muscle mass, but many of them now had joint problems and difficulty walking. He didn't know much about factory farming, but he knew artificially supported growth when he saw it. He recognized what happens when short-term bulk matters and long-term consequences don't.

Like this man's football teammates, modern pigs' growth and "performance" are unnaturally enhanced. The pigs at Farm Sanctuary are on a special high-fiber vegan feed, but it's still hard to manage their weight as they get older. Many develop leg or foot ailments. It's sad. Because many of the older pigs have trouble standing, they spend much of their time lying down. Mornings are when they are the most active, since it's cooler then. In the afternoons, you'll usually find the pigs taking long siestas.

If the pigs at our shelters hadn't been rescued, they wouldn't have lived beyond about six months and 250 pounds. I feel good about the fact that we've given them a longer life in a more natural setting. But they have been engineered to industry specifications, so we can only help so much. When the older pigs, usually around eight or nine years, start to have trouble moving around, we are faced with a painful decision: is euthanasia more humane than keeping them alive and so weighed down? It's never an easy answer.

Indoctrination

Pigmanship. Surely one aspect of its meaning must be a certain empathy with the animal—an acknowledgment that he or she has needs and wants. How, then, can people who should know better create a life of such unrelieved misery for pigs and other farmed animals? I found the answer in the first few weeks of my time at Cornell University's School of Agriculture and Life Sciences.

Cornell is both a land grant university and a member of the Ivy League. It is conveniently close to the Watkins Glen shelter, and I thought that earning a degree from the school would provide me with useful information about current agricultural practices and would complement my independent reading of agribusiness journals. The program would also, I thought, help me to understand the mind-set of people going into farming today. Cornell is held in high esteem by agriculturalists, so having a master's degree in agricultural economics from there would give me some credibility in my encounters with farmers and help open doors. And it has.

During my two years at Cornell, I took courses in animal science, economics, and rural sociology. My fellow students were fairly mixed, half men and half women. Many wanted to become veterinarians. On the first day of an animal science class, the professor spent some time warning us about animal rights activists and how these ill-intended individuals might be seen lurking around the animal barns on campus. If a student saw anyone fitting this description, the professor said, he or she should report that person to the authorities. No one in the program knew I was a vegan animal advocate who ran a sanctuary about forty-five minutes away, and I was in no hurry to clue them in, especially since I'd just been warned to watch out for myself!

My freshman animal science class gave me firsthand experience of the desensitization and acculturation students go through as they pursue careers in animal agriculture. Cornell has a small swine unit, located in a barn close to the main campus. After class, we could walk over to the building and see the pigs. The sows were kept in farrowing crates. One day the class gathered around two crates, each with a sow and about ten newborn piglets. A graduate student had been assigned to teach us several routine farming procedures.

The first was tail docking, a practice, he explained, that was done to stop the pigs from gnawing one another's tails. Tail biting, as it is called, is an unhealthy behavior that occurs when pigs are crowded in barren enclosures. Our confident teacher picked up one of the piglets and, using a tool that looked like a pair of pliers, grabbed the piglet's tail. As he squeezed the handle, he yanked the piglet's body away, ripping the tail off and leaving a bleeding stump. The tiny piglet screamed.

The graduate student next demonstrated what he called ear notching. This, he explained, was necessary so the animals could be identified. This involved cutting triangular chunks of skin out of the piglets' ears with an instrument designed for the purpose. The student told us he recommended cutting the notches deep since that made it easier to recognize the animals. He then began to cut each piglet's ear multiple times. With each cut, the piglets would struggle and squeal. By the time he was finished, the piglets were bleeding profusely and blood covered the floor.

I looked at my fellow students. Many of them were visibly squeamish. Several turned away or avoided his gaze when the graduate student encouraged the class to try their hand at cutting off a piglet's tail or notching an ear. He was very persistent, as well as confident and self-assured. Eventually, a young man stepped forward and was coached in mutilating the piglet while the rest of us looked on. A second student followed. Each time a new student came forward, I could see the group's initial resistance draining away. Eventually, most stopped turning away or looking down, and they began accepting these practices as normal.

A day after the piglet mutilation, we returned to the farrowing crates and found most of the piglets gone. They had bled to death. Our instructor explained that their deaths were the result of a genetic defect. The company that had provided the sows, the Pig Improvement Company (PIC), had been notified so the problem could be fixed. Not once did we discuss the possibility that our carving up of these newborns' ears or cutting off their tails might have been responsible for their deaths. It was the victims' fault, not ours.

In the early 1960s, the scientist Stanley Milgram conducted a set of experiments at Yale University that showed how ordinary people could overcome their resistance to harming others when they were assured by a figure in authority—in this case, a scientist—that he would take responsibility for whatever happened and that what they were asked to do was necessary and useful. Milgram employed actors to mimic the effects of an electric shock and told the participating individuals to turn a dial that would send larger and larger amounts of "electricity" to shock the subject. These ordinary residents of New Haven, Connecticut, were unaware that the subjects were actors and that no electric current was in use.

As the participants turned the dial, the actor displayed ever-increasing amounts of "pain," and the person controlling the dial became more and more distressed. Each time, the scientist assured him or her that what was happening was okay. What astounded Milgram was that almost two-thirds of the people in the study were willing to inflict significant pain—simulated shocks of up to 450 volts—despite their instinctual discomfort, and for no reason other than that a scientist had told them to. When they were made public, the results of the experiments scandalized the country.

I saw a similar mind-set on display in that class at Cornell: a resistance to asking questions, a desire to fit in with others, and an ability to suppress feelings of anguish or empathy if either got in the way of pleasing a trusted authority. In this way, we can develop behaviors and habits that become the unquestioned norm. The great nineteenth-century environmental writer and philosopher Henry David Thoreau summed up this phenomenon in *Walden:* "It is remarkable how easily and insensibly we fall into a particular route, and make a beaten track for ourselves. . . . The surface of the earth is soft and impressionable by the feet of men; and so with the paths which the mind travels. How worn and dusty, then, must be the highways of the world, how deep the ruts of tradition and conformity!"

I would like to believe that what happened that day in the animal science class caused some of the students to question standard practices that left animals suffering in their blood-soaked pens. Instead, I'm afraid it simply reinforced the notion that humans have the ability, and even a duty, to use animals for our purposes, without constraint. Any negative consequences were not our fault, but the result of a malfunctioning but fixable technology.

Trying to fix animals to suit our purposes has become a matter for the lab scientists. Despite a growing recognition that pigs and other farm animals are intelligent and social creatures, the majority of industry-related research continues to focus on developing profitable and expedient animal production methods. Feed is among the food animal industry's greatest input costs, so land grant university scientists have conducted enormous amounts of research into how to most efficiently and cheaply feed pigs to bring them to market. Pigs are fattened on corn-based, drug-laced food designed to achieve maximum growth at minimal cost.

In response to concerns about human obesity and the large amount of fat in the average American's diet, scientists have genetically engineered leaner pigs. Unfortunately, leaner pigs suffer from increased levels of stress, a problem so common that it has been given a name: porcine stress syndrome, or PSS. During my time at Cornell I recall a boar dubbed "Arnold Schwarzenegger" because he was so muscular. He was big, all right—and so high-strung that he would nearly pass out from the stress of mating.

Citizen Initiative

In 2002 Farm Sanctuary and other groups and individuals ran a campaign to ban gestation crates in Florida. Efforts to get a federal law passed that would end the use of these and other cruel factory farming devices haven't yet met with success, but we have made progress with statewide efforts to regulate conditions for farmed animals.

During my research for the campaign, I visited two facilities owned by the same man. Conditions at the first farm couldn't have been more shocking. In the fattening barn, I came across a couple of pens full of living, dying, and dead pigs, some of whom had been partially consumed by the others. It seemed as though the farmer had simply dumped the sick pigs there to fend for themselves. The barn was so littered with bones and other parts of dead pigs that it was impossible to avoid stepping on them. I remember feeling the desperation of one terrified downed pig who shook with spasms as she lay on the brink of death and being eaten. This grisly scene gave new meaning to the notion of a dog-eat-dog, or in this case pig-eat-pig, world.

At the second facility, I observed a level of sensitivity toward the pigs.

After years of confinement the pigs' muscles had atrophied and they had a variety of health problems. As a remedy, the farmer put up a temporary fence around a field and allowed the sows outdoors to walk, root, and graze on the corn stubble. At another Florida pig farm, I saw sows who had recently given birth living with their piglets, and I watched as they interacted with one another and wandered around a wooded area. The piglets followed their mothers around, and the mothers nuzzled and guided them. This farm had a sense of calm and community unlike any industrialized farm I'd ever visited.

Back in the year 2000, a number of groups concerned about the welfare of farmed animals, including Farm Sanctuary, tried to ban gestation crates through the Florida legislature. A bill was introduced, but it was referred to the agriculture committee of the state's assembly and died without getting a hearing. That pig farmer I'd met was right: it wasn't hard to kill a bill in Tallahassee. This didn't really surprise us, since agriculture committees are almost always made up of legislators friendly to agribusiness interests.

Since Florida was one of twenty or so states with a process in place to get initiatives on the ballot, Farm Sanctuary, along with the Animal Rights Foundation of Florida and the Humane Society of the United States, decided to go directly to the people and collect the necessary signatures to put a measure banning gestation crates before the voters in the November 2002 elections. We didn't get all the allies we'd expected or hoped for. That summer, the American Veterinary Medical Association, which we thought would support the ballot initiative, passed a resolution at its annual meeting stating that gestation crates were an appropriate way to house sows. Those of us on the ground in Florida found ourselves having to explain that the veterinary association was representing the interests of industrial farming rather than the animals themselves. (Unfortunately, the AVMA has barely changed its attitudes since then. It has failed to adopt various resolutions promoting basic farmed animal welfare.)

In spite of the major blow from the AVMA that industry hoped would derail the initiative, voters came through. When they cast their ballots in November 2002, 55 percent of Floridians voted to add language to the state constitution to ban gestation crates. The ban, going into effect in 2008, gave farmers using the crates time to develop alternatives.

Within a few months, a few farmers sold their pigs and made the ridiculous claim that even though it would be six years before the ban would take effect, they'd been effectively forced out of business. It wasn't true, but it was a convenient story for many farmers resistant to animal welfare. This account, manufactured though it was, led to a bill being introduced in the Florida state legislature that would have given these two farmers several hundred thousand dollars to ease their supposed hardship. The bill was passed by both chambers, then vetoed by Florida governor Jeb Bush, who must have seen it for what it was: pork.

The legislature wasn't finished. Another bill was introduced that would have amended and removed certain provisions of the state constitution, tidied up the language, and taken away some of the initiatives that had been passed. This bill earmarked about six initiatives to be removed and placed in statute, where they could be more easily changed by the legislature. One by one the groups that advocated for the initiatives were able to get them taken out of the legislation, until the gestation crate ban was the only one left. Given the history of the Florida legislature, we were more than a little concerned. Fortunately, time ran out and the effort to remove the initiative from the constitution was defeated.

I hope that the passing of the ban will lead to many other state bans, and then perhaps a broader campaign to challenge common farming practices that are inhumane, unethical, and inappropriate. But it will not be easy. With each victory our opposition is becoming increasingly organized and clever in its efforts to fight change.

In E. B. White's classic children's book *Charlotte's Web*, a young girl, Fern, grows attached to her pig, Wilbur. When Wilbur is moved to her uncle Homer Zuckerman's farm to be fattened for slaughter, he's lonely and scared until he meets Charlotte, a barnyard spider. Charlotte recognizes Wilbur's individuality, and spins strange and wonderful words such as "Some Pig" into her web in an effort to save his life. It works, and Wilbur becomes the toast of the countryside. White himself raised animals on his farm in Maine, and apparently his own struggle with slaughtering a pig who'd become a friend inspired *Charlotte's Web*.

Like the fictional farmer Zuckerman, White spared his pig the chopping block. In an essay about this experience he wrote: "I began to feel sorry for the pig because, like most pigs, he was doomed. This made me sad, so I started thinking of ways to save a pig's life." I'm very glad he did. His book, which a grammar school teacher read to my class, has inspired generations of children to look at farmed animals (as well as spiders, of course) with fresh eyes.

What I have discovered from the tiny fraction of a percent of U.S. farmed animals that Farm Sanctuary has sheltered over the years is that each of them—no matter how commodified or denatured by the industry—is, like Wilbur, an individual. Each one has a distinct personality as well as his or her own needs, fears, and desire to live. Every one of them who dies in our factory farms and slaughterhouses was, as White wrote, a creature who "had suffered in a suffering world."

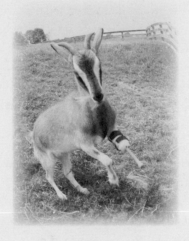

Zoop

PROFILE: ZOOP

Goat's meat and milk are consumed by people around the world. While neither is a mainstream staple in the U.S. diet, growing demand from Latin American, Caribbean, and Muslim communities is driving up the numbers of goats raised for slaughter. Between 1999 and 2005, goat meat consumption in the United States rose by a whopping 64 percent, and it's expected to grow by roughly 10 percent a year. About two million goats are currently being raised in the United States for meat. An additional half a million are farmed for milk and mohair (the latter are usually sold for meat in the end, too). Like other livestock raised for slaughter, goats may be kept on the range, where they aren't adequately protected from extreme weather conditions, or confined in feedlots, where they often fall prey to respiratory ailments common to filthy, crowded pens.

A relatively large number of goats are killed in accordance with ritual laws—for example, halal or kosher slaughter. This requires the animals to be fully conscious, often hanging by a back leg, while their throats are cut. Many goats are killed by custom-exempt operations that are not covered by the Humane Slaughter Act. Growing demand for halal meat has led to the spread of urban live meat markets—and a consequent rise in the number of abandoned or runaway goats loose on city streets. Zoop was one of those runaways, a rust-colored goat with white stripes on her face and a white belly. She was found in Denville, New Jersey, in a snowstorm, walking on her knees, a six-pound baby at the time. She must have been dumped, perhaps by a live market that didn't want to deal with her injured legs. A kind law enforcement officer took Zoop to a nearby animal hospital, which gave her a brace for one leg and did surgery to try to repair the other.

After six months, Zoop came to our Watkins Glen shelter, where she could be around other goats and live on a pasture. She fit right in. Goats are very social, and if you separate one from the others, you can count on some vocal protests. (Incidentally, goats and sheep also get along well. In fact, at Watkins Glen, we have special-needs goats who live with the sheep. One, Dino, seems to think he is a sheep.) Zoop became close with Juniper, another rescued goat who struggles with leg problems. Unfortunately, Zoop didn't heal as well as we'd hoped, and the vets at Cornell ultimately determined that one of her legs was so damaged that it had to be amputated above the knee. After recovering from the surgery, Zoop was fitted with a prosthetic leg. With her new leg, her mobility has increased dramatically and her spirits are higher than ever. Now Zoop is walking and running and butting heads (she likes to play rough), and even the most ambitious goats in our herd have trouble keeping up.

Texas is the leading goat-producing state, followed by Tennessee and California. The New Holland stockyard near Lancaster, Pennsylvania, is a big seller of goats for ethnic markets. At this writing the domestic supply cannot meet the demand, so the United States imports more than seventeen million pounds of goat meat each year from Australia and New Zealand.

As with all animals seen as units of production, abuses in the U.S. goat industry are not uncommon. Two recent cases are particularly shocking, and I'm glad to report both resulted in legal action. In 2004, the head of a dairy goat association was charged with mistreating animals for allegedly killing kids, as baby goats are known, with a claw hammer, performing a cesarean section on a pregnant goat with no anesthesia, and setting a goat on fire before cutting the animal's throat. That same year, Farm Sanctuary uncovered a Wisconsin farm where countless dead goats were piled amid live animals, without food or water. Twenty-six of the goats were brought to our Watkins Glen shelter, where they received emergency veterinary care and rehabilitation. In this case, the farm's owner was charged with twenty counts of animal cruelty.

CHAPTER TEN

The Pecking Disorder

If playground name-calling is any indication, we humans hold birds in pretty low regard. The cowardly or stupid are "chickens" or "turkeys," the forgetful or dumb "birdbrained." We refer to an oft-nagged friend as "henpecked." Why birds are held in such low esteem is a bit of a mystery to me. Perhaps it's because they look so different from us. They're not mammals, after all, and their feathers and beaks (and in some cases their wattles or combs or snoods) may put that much more distance between us. Perhaps we make assumptions about birds because we really don't know them. But a growing body of research is shedding new light on the intelligence of birds and their cognitive abilities. There's even an argument to be made that calling someone a birdbrain is a compliment.

But none of that saves them from slaughter. Over the past two decades, the number of chickens raised for human consumption in the United States has increased substantially, from 6 billion to around 8.7 billion, and as of this writing it's still on the rise. It's a colossal number—almost beyond imagining. Yet, before these chickens are turned into nuggets or drumsticks, breasts or wings, they are living, feeling animals with hearts, brains, and a desire to live. When they die, they die one by one, as individuals, not inventory.

Fifty years of industrial farming cannot stop the millions of years of evolution that shaped them into complex and fascinating creatures. Hens and roosters, for instance, form flocks or family units, usually with one rooster and several hens. Some chicken family groups do have two roosters, but that's not the norm since the males tend to compete. The roosters operate according to a chivalric code of sorts. They watch out for the hens and shelter them from danger, including predators, and alert them to happy news, too, like the arrival of a new supply of tasty food. The birds may peck each other, but mostly in a friendly way. They're grooming, clearing mites and parasites from one another's feathers. Most roosters aren't unreconstructed patriarchs. They let the hens eat first. But if there's a hawk in the area, they'll warn the hens and make sure they get to safety. We even had one rooster who died in an attempt to protect his hens from a hawk attack.

At the Orland shelter, we have a number of blind hens, and the roosters who live with them are really their lifeline, making sure they know where to eat, sleep, and roost. Most traditional farmers have a soft spot for roosters. They're invaluable additions to a flock and to the farm. One such individual was Purdie, a chick I rescued from a hatchery and raised in the house. We enjoyed each other's company, and he and I would greet each other when I came home. When Purdie grew older, I put him out in the barn with the other chickens, and for weeks he tried to convince me that he was really a part of my flock, running over to me whenever I approached. Finally, he got used to his new chicken family and was at home among his "people."

Even if they've known only factory farm conditions before they come to us, hens quickly learn to enjoy straw and use it to build nests. They like privacy when they're laying eggs, and so we have nest boxes at our shelters. Hens also have pecking orders. They'll fight among themselves to work things out, but then make up. In general, chickens are very social. They enjoy each other's company and they're often curious about people. What always amazes me is how quickly factory-farmed chickens remember how to be chickens. Even if they've never set foot outside a cage or been outdoors, almost immediately after they arrive at Farm Sanctuary they're walking, unsteadily at first, but then with confidence. Soon they're exploring their new surroundings, pecking at the earth, spreading and flapping their wings, and taking dust baths. Their resilience inspires me.

Inside a Chicken Factory Farm

Chicken farming in the United States consists of raising two distinct strains of domestic chickens. Broilers are those raised for meat, and layers are raised to lay eggs. Broilers have been selectively bred to grow twice as fast and twice as large as normal, while laying hens have been genetically selected to efficiently convert the calories they get from feed into egg production. By contrast with the broilers, egg-laying hens do not grow very fast or large.

The life of a commercial chicken begins at the hatchery, where fertilized eggs are placed in drawers stacked in ceiling-high incubators resembling massive industrial refrigerators. Temperature and humidity are carefully controlled and monitored, and after about three weeks the chicks peck their way out of their shells. They are then removed from the incubators, and a machine separates any partially hatched chicks from their eggshells. Like any machine, this one can malfunction, but in this case the cost is lives—many a frail young bird is dismembered in the process. The survivors are moved to their various destinations quickly, in crates and on conveyor belts, and handled more or less like tomatoes as line workers sort the hatchlings by sex.

In order to reduce injuries from pecking, female chicks earmarked to become egg-laying hens are debeaked soon after hatching. This involves cutting off part of the bird's sensitive beak and is performed without anesthesia. It is painful and at times fatal. At hatcheries that produce laying hens, the males, approximately half of the hatchlings, are of no use. They don't grow fast enough to be raised profitably for meat and will never lay eggs, so they—along with the weak, injured, or deformed chicks—are simply discarded.

How best to dispose of these unwanted male chicks has puzzled modern industrial farming for years. Approximately 300 million layer hens are used in commercial egg production in the United States. For each of them, there was once a corresponding and unwanted male chick. After extensive research, the animal scientists determined that one of the most "humane" and efficient ways to kill these millions of male chicks is high-speed maceration. This involves dumping the live chicks into a machine where they quickly meet with its whirring blades. It doesn't take long to turn them into fertilizer or chicken feed. When I first started researching this issue, I called the USDA and asked for recommendations on how to dispose of chicks. Their advice: buy an industrial garbage disposal like those used in commercial kitchen sinks.

Like other practices employed by the industry for speed and expedited production, the maceration machine is not perfect. When it malfunctions or too many chicks are loaded too quickly, the blades slow or jam, and live birds are chopped up piece by piece rather than killed swiftly in the oversized blender. Unbelievably grisly as it is, other methods (such as suffocation or gassing) may be worse. But humane or not, maceration is an economically viable way to turn a liability (male chicks) into a sellable asset (chicken feed), and so it's become a standard industry practice.

The gruesome things I've seen on my visits to hatcheries over the years will stay with me for the rest of my life: a worker shoveling "garbage," which included live and dead chicks along with eggshells and other debris, into a dumpster; thousands of male chicks in trash cans and plastic bags, suffocated under the weight of others piled on top of them; a hatchling fighting his way out from the bottom of a clear plastic garbage bag, scrambling over weak and dead baby birds to escape; that same chick in a large dumpster, standing and chirping his disorientation amid thousands of dead and discarded chicks.

I have watched unwanted chicks dumped onto an auger, a large screwlike device that is customarily used for processing grain or sand, then dropped through an opening in the side of the building into a manure spreader outside. I could hear faint chirping as live chicks, many of them horribly injured, were ground up and their feathers, flesh, and blood deposited on cropland as fertilizer. I later walked the field looking for survivors but found only mangled, lifeless bodies among the corn stubble. What stays with me most is the terrible irony of these newly hatched chicks, symbols of spring and rebirth, who'd been driven to fight their way out of their shell by the instinct to live that we all share, only to be ground up alive and turned into manure. And all because, in the industry's eyes, they have no value.

Unlike the egg industry, the broiler industry uses both female and male birds: 8.7 billion of them are raised for meat every year in the United States. The young chicks destined to be broilers move along a conveyor belt into chambers where a mist administers the vaccinations they will need to help survive the factory farm diseases that await them. The broilers are crowded into massive sheds called grower houses that commonly contain tens of thousands of birds. They aren't kept in cages, living instead on the shed floor, but that doesn't mean they have much room to move. Each bird is allotted about half a square foot of space, though in a matter of weeks they will weigh around five pounds.

What first strikes you when you step inside these facilities is the smell. The air is so dense with the ammonia produced by the chickens' feces that your eyes tear up and your lungs feel as though they're burning. The chickens form a vast sea of white feathers rippling nervously away from you as you enter. But because the birds are so densely packed they can barely move without pressing against each other.

For the duration of their time in the grower houses, the chickens are supplied with feed laced with growth-enhancing drugs and chemicals, including arsenic (a known carcinogen that is in most forms toxic) delivered through automated feed troughs that run the length of the buildings. The goal is to make food readily available to the fast-growing birds. Artificial lighting stimulates the birds to consume more, grow fast, and reach market weight as quickly as possible. The birds have been genetically manipulated to develop extra-large breasts, the part of their body that consumers prefer. The poultry industry boasts about the fact that it takes only forty-two days to bring a five- to six-pound chicken to market—fifty years ago it took more than three months.

Unfortunately, this massive jump in growth rates has had severe consequences for animal welfare. The most obvious is the poor health of the birds. They grow so fast and large that their hearts and lungs can't keep pace, and every year millions of these young birds die of heart failure before reaching slaughter weight. Inside grower houses you see birds who've died and others barely able to walk. Birds keeling over and dying is so common that there's a name for it—it's called flip-over syndrome. Flip-over is virtually unheard of among farmers who breed and raise chickens naturally, with more space and healthier food.

The ammonia in bird feces affects the birds as well, and it's not hard to find a few gasping for air on the shed floor. Studies have shown that factory-farmed birds experience respiratory problems, including infectious bronchitis, while workers are at risk for bronchitis, occupational asthma, and long-term lung damage. The birds receive little human care or attention except when a worker comes through the building to remove dead and dying birds, or when they are taken to slaughter. Truly, the air can be so noxious that no one would go into a grower house unless he or she had to. The birds, on the other hand, don't have a choice.

The air quality is not the only problem. The floor in grower houses is usually covered with litter made of wood shavings. Because the litter is not changed regularly, it becomes progressively more and more soiled with waste, burning the birds' feet, legs, and chests. The chickens' unbalanced and heavy bodies place an enormous strain on their legs and joints, causing crippling lameness and further increasing the risk of burns. In the United States, where agribusiness is careful to conceal such blemishes from consumers, damaged bird parts are ground up into processed foods where they go unnoticed.

Because the economic benefits of the modern approach to raising chickens outweigh the costs, it is possible for farmers to absorb enormous losses of life. A chicken can be worth less than a dollar to the producer, which means that treating sick birds is just not worth it; it's cheaper to let them die and then restock. While poultry industry veterinarians do perform necropsies to see whether a bird died of a transmissible disease, they aren't interested in the welfare of individual animals. Their concern is preventing the spread of an infection through the flock and the subsequent loss of revenues.

Chickens, like other animals, need to fulfill their instincts. They require fresh air, sunlight, and grass, and in factory sheds they are denied all of these. A normal social group would consist of about twenty birds, but in factory farming situations chickens can't develop the complex system of hierarchy and relationships that we know proverbially as a pecking order. Even so, they try. Observant farmers have noticed chickens in grower houses moving together in smaller groups among the flock, possibly trying to create a normal-size social system. I have seen birds try to satisfy their perching instinct by sitting awkwardly on top of feeding equipment. Others engage in dust bathing to help control lice—but in grower houses, of course, the dirt consists of litter soaked in waste.

When the broiler chickens reach slaughter weight, a group of what are called catchers, usually young men, grab the birds by the legs, five or six to a hand, and sling them from the shed into transport crates. As one building is emptied, the catchers move on to the next. It is backbreaking labor for markedly low wages: for each thousand birds, workers are paid about two dollars. The pressure to move at a good clip is an enormous strain on the workers, and they often take their stress and frustration out on the birds. Studies have shown that large numbers of birds are injured in the move from shed to transport crate to slaughter. Attempting to lessen the problem (read: something that cuts into profits), the industry is beginning to offer more money to workers who can limit the number of birds who arrive at the slaughterhouse dead.

As befitting the term *factory* farming, a machine has been developed to replace the chicken catchers. It looks like a crop harvester, with a wide front area that collects the birds and funnels them into the crates. I understand the benefits of using machinery to relieve humans of hard labor. (I was a very happy man when we got our first tractor to help carry feed, fence posts, and other heavy items around the farm.) But the main goal of this particular innovation is not to save the backs of the workers; it's to cut costs even further. Neither human nor machine can humanely catch birds at the rate expected on today's farms. And because the system is overloaded, problems inevitably arise. It is likely that if the catching machines became standard, the whole frightening process—and its attendant losses—would just kick up into a higher gear.

Believe it or not the life of a layer hen is even worse. In fact, in terms of the intensity and length of their confinement, chickens used for egg production are perhaps the most abused of all farm animals. Three hundred million layer hens in the United States produce the eggs we eat. They spend their lives in "battery" cages (thus named in reference to the vast battery of cages) that are lined up in rows and stacked in tiers in huge warehouses that can each contain more than eighty thousand birds. These realities are not widely known to consumers, many of whom believe they're reducing animal suffering when they choose eggs instead of meat.

The hens are commonly packed six or eight to a cage that is all of twenty inches wide. In other words, each bird can barely move and lives in a space less than the length and width of a sheet of 8½-by-11-inch paper. The hens' feed is mechanically delivered to a trough at the front of the cage. The floors of the cages are made of wire, which expedites egg collection and manure removal but contributes to broken bones, foot and leg injuries, and severe pain for the hens. Their feces drop through the wire cages, but there's no way for the hens to rest comfortably, even when they are laying eggs. The cage floors are also set on an angle, so gravity does the work of collecting the eggs (they roll onto conveyor belts), another example of production goals trumping animal welfare concerns. In short, the cages are a constant source of discomfort for the hens.

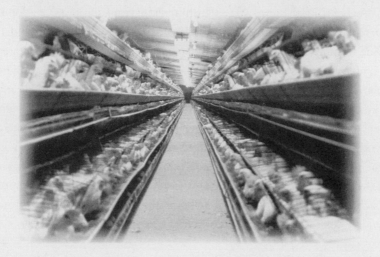

Battery cages

With the hens packed tightly and pushing constantly against the sides of their cages, a hen's legs, head, and wings can become entangled in the wire, causing injury or, if she can't reach food or water, death. Unlike the broilers, the layers are kept in sheds that are dimly lit, to keep chickens less active than they would be outside. That means they require less feed and are less likely to damage themselves as they move and rub against the wire boundaries of the cage. Even so, many battery-caged chickens endure bruises, abrasions, and severe feather loss.

Even more constrained than their broiler cousins, battery-caged hens cannot walk, exercise, forage, or peck the ground in search of bugs or seeds. They cannot stretch or flap their wings, or preen and ruffle their feathers. They cannot build nests or find a small private area to lay their eggs, as they would in more natural surroundings. Unable to fulfill their most basic needs, the hens experience extreme frustration and have no outlet for their aggression other than to peck each other. This is why the industry insists on debeaking them.

Over the years Farm Sanctuary has catalogued the cruelties of the egg industry and sought to educate the public about the wretched lives of layer hens. We have also advocated that battery cages be outlawed in the United States, as they have been in parts of Europe. While there are moves to increase the space allotted to caged layers in the United States from forty-eight to sixty-seven square inches, the increase would only marginally improve the hens' welfare and do little to reduce their physical and psychological discomfort.

I have been inside many of these layer hen facilities. The buildings are commonly two stories tall with narrow catwalks in between long rows of battery cages. The entire first floor is waste storage. In addition to chicken manure, the floor is covered with tattered feathers, broken eggs, bodies, and live birds who have fallen or escaped from their cages. Some die of starvation, drown, or suffocate in a putrid ocean of their own waste. On more than one occasion, I have found myself wading through this ocean, trying to help the trapped birds. Walking through the muck, I have felt the crunch of bones under my feet; I was too late for those already dead birds. Because my purpose is not immediately obvious to the desperate hens and my boots are encrusted in manure, hens who are able to scurry away do so. It's usually only possible to rescue the sick and dying.

Not long ago, we took in hens from a battery cage egg farm run by Wegmans, an upstate New York supermarket chain known for its generally progressive business model. The hens had been wandering in the manure pit for some time, and they had tennis-ball-sized clumps of manure caked onto their feet. When they got to Farm Sanctuary, the shelter staff had to cut away the encrusted manure and feathers. We could see that the hens' feet were atrophied, because they'd been encased in that hardened muck for so long. That didn't stop them from taking their first few steps just a few minutes later, as soon as they hit the straw on the barn floor. Their claws were weak, but their will was strong.

Over the last several decades, layer hens' bodies have been profoundly manipulated and pushed to produce an extraordinary 265 eggs a year, many times the number they would naturally lay. As with other high-performance farmed animals, this level of productivity puts an enormous strain on the hens' bodies. According to an article in *Lancaster Farming* newspaper, the amount of calcium used to produce the shells of the eggs over the course of a year is thirty times the weight of the hen's skeleton, which means the hens are chronically depleted of calcium. As in people, this deficiency leads to osteoporosis and other conditions such as the potentially fatal cage layer fatigue. The hens can also die of egg-bound syndrome, when their overworked bodies cannot expel another egg and become clogged. Over the years, Farm Sanctuary has rescued thousands of former egg-laying hens, and many have eventually succumbed to this condition.

In a natural setting, hens can live more than ten years. However, after a year in the battery cages, the hen's productivity begins to drop off, which means she is no longer useful to the industry. So, like a worn-out piece of machinery, she's replaced. Before she is, however, she may be put through one more arduous production cycle. If she isn't sent to slaughter immediately, the hen could go through what's called force-molting, a common industry practice. Hens are starved for up to two weeks in order to shock their bodies into a new egg-laying cycle—they get no reward or respite. After McDonald's, Burger King, and Wendy's refused to buy eggs from hens who were force-molted, factory farms are phasing out the practice of starving hens, but they may still trigger a molt, and another egg production cycle, with a nutrient-deficient diet.

After about a year, or two if they are force-molted, the laying hens are considered "spent" and are shipped to slaughter, where their bruised and battered bodies can be ground up or shredded to make low-grade meat products such as chicken soup or potpie. There's not much meat on these thin, old layers, and it's become increasingly difficult to find slaughterhouses willing to take them. Why would they when there's a ready supply of heavy, meaty broiler chickens available? An egg farmer in upstate New York told me he had to send his spent hens to Canada to be slaughtered. Other factory farmers take more extreme measures. One battery cage facility operator in southern California who wanted to dispose of thirty thousand unwanted laying hens came up with a resourceful solution: he put them into a wood chipper. Neighbors were horrified to see live birds being fed into the chipper and reported it to local authorities, who charged the egg farmer with cruelty to animals. The charges were ultimately dropped, however, because a poultry industry veterinarian—yes, you read that right, a *veterinarian*—gave his considered opinion that the wood chipper was an acceptable method for disposing of live birds.

Modern Times in a Poultry Slaughterhouse

The process of factory-farming animals reminds me of Charlie Chaplin's film *Modern Times*, the 1930s satire on the soullessness of industrialization. Like the farmers and the workers in slaughterhouses, Chaplin fails to keep up with the factory line's never-ending supply of bolts that he is charged with tightening. Chaplin's character is pushed to the limit and finally, unable to cope, is caught in the very machine he's trying to service. Chaplin plays it for the laugh and it is funny, but in the life-and-death scenario of the slaughterhouse there's little comic relief. Indeed, mechanized, industrialized farming has served to desensitize us, making it easier to raise and kill animals by the billions. Speed and mechanization aid our callousness: it's easier to perpetrate violence and harm when we see neither the faces of our victims nor the painful effects of our actions. And nowhere in industrial farming is this heartlessness clearer than at a poultry slaughterhouse.

Many people assume there are regulations or laws in place to ensure that farmed animals' deaths are painless and quick. In fact, the federal Humane Methods of Slaughter Act has numerous limitations. Most startlingly, it had been interpreted to exempt poultry from its provisions entirely, even though birds account for more than *95 percent* of all the animals killed for food in the United States. No reasonable justification exists for this.

At a poultry slaughterhouse, a forklift or similar machine removes transport crates from the truck and tilts them over a conveyor belt, and out fall the chickens. One after another, crateloads of birds spill onto a conveyor, where some break bones or miss the belt entirely and land on the floor, where they are often run over by machinery. The scale is breathtaking. One slaughter plant can unload and kill more than five thousand birds an hour per slaughter line. Workers lift conscious birds by their legs and hook their feet into shackles at a rate of eighteen hundred birds an hour, or about one bird every two seconds. Like Chaplin's Little Tramp, line workers have difficulty maintaining this speed, and many suffer from back injuries or cumulative trauma disorders. The compromised well-being of workers seriously impairs their ability to lift the birds humanely.

Once shackled, the chickens travel along the rail to a stunning tank, where their heads pass through a tank of electrified water. The current is meant to immobilize the birds in order to facilitate rapid and efficient killing. However, the jolt is not sufficient to ensure that the birds are insensible to pain, and they can remain conscious, though paralyzed, as they continue on the disassembly line.

After the stunning tank, the birds come to a mechanical blade that cuts their throats, one after another in rapid succession. It's about speed, not accuracy, and sometimes the blade misses entirely or injures the birds without killing them. Workers are stationed and ready to manually slit the throats of birds that escape death by the mechanical blade. However, the line moves so fast that workers often can't keep up.

The next stage is the scalding tank, where the birds are submerged in boiling water to loosen their feathers. By then, they are supposed to have bled to death but, incredibly, some are still alive and conscious. USDA records show that millions of chickens are boiled alive every year.

After the scalding tank, the birds' feathers, heads, and innards are removed and their bodies are cut up. They are eventually packaged whole or as breasts, legs, or other component parts and then refrigerated and shipped out to wholesale and retail markets. Damaged birds and those whose body parts are not suitable for display in clear plastic are further processed, ground up into nuggets and other products where the birds' damaged bodies will go unnoticed.

Disease and contamination also go unnoticed. The USDA's Food Safety and Inspection Service has found that 16 percent of broiler chickens in the United States are now contaminated with salmonella, up from 9 percent in 2000. Tyson, Pilgrim's Pride, and Perdue were among the agribusiness giants whose broiler chicken processing plants failed to meet the USDA's standard for salmonella contamination at least once between January 1998 and December 2005. There are over a million cases of salmonellosis (infection with the salmonella bacteria) each year in the

United States tied to eating meat and poultry. According to the USDA, 9,000 victims have to be hospitalized and more than 250 of them die. The USDA estimates that the cost of illness and premature death from salmonella each year is $1.5 billion.

Virgil Butler made his living in surroundings like I've just described. A native of rural Arkansas, he got his first job at age fourteen, catching chickens in grower sheds at night. He attended high school during the day, and the demands of his schedule and the unhealthy conditions at work soon took a physical toll. "There was rarely a night that I went home and didn't have a screaming backache. My hands would swell until they looked like baseball gloves," he said.

When he was older, Butler took on various jobs at chicken slaughter-houses, sometimes hanging the birds in the metal shackles, sometimes slitting the throats of the birds that the machines missed. At first, the killing bothered him. "The chickens were hanging there in those shackles, helpless. To me, it was extremely unfair simply because they were so innocent."

Butler saw the inadequacy of the killing process firsthand. "It really bothered me when I missed one and heard the poor bird go through the scalder alive, thrashing and bumping against the sides as it slowly died. I worked to become really good at killing so that I wouldn't miss so many. I did become really good, but at a steep price. The more I did it, the less it bothered me. I became desensitized. The killing room really does something to your mind—all that blood, killing so many times, over and over again. Working as a killer was what I hated the most."

Other slaughterhouse workers went through that same desensitization process, and some began to treat the birds with cruelty and contempt. "I have seen [co-workers] shove dry ice up the rectums of chickens to blow them up. I have seen them stuff the head of one inside the rectum of another and so on, making a kind of 'train' of birds. I have seen people bash the birds against the belt, throw them into walls, stomp them, throw them into fans, squeeze them so hard that they would spray feces all over another worker (you could hear the bones pop in their rib cages when they did this). These are just some of the little 'games' people would play." According to Butler, who became an anti-factory-farming activist, the violence extended beyond the slaughterhouse: "Other co-workers became violent toward their own families. The longer I worked there, the more violent I became. Life became meaningless—other people's lives became meaningless. I got to thinking that if I had this ability to kill and not care, then the same thing was happening to the others. I trusted no one." Sadly, Virgil died at the end of 2006. As one of the few slaughter-house workers willing to speak out against factory farming cruelty, his voice will be greatly missed.

America's Respectable Bird

In January 1784, Benjamin Franklin sent a letter to his daughter from France criticizing the decision to make the bald eagle the symbol of the fledgling American republic. "He is a Bird of bad Moral Character," wrote Franklin about the bald eagle. "He does not get his living honestly. . . . [T]he Turkey is in Comparison a much more respectable Bird, and withal a true original Native of America." In Franklin's time, slender, bronze-colored, swift wild turkeys were abundant. Today, wild turkeys are much less common, although you can still find them in wooded parts of North America, foraging for seeds and insects and sleeping in the low branches of trees at night. Though many people don't know this, wild turkeys can fly.

Turkeys raised for food in the United States bear little resemblance to their wild cousins. They have been bred to be white, because the plumage of darker breeds leaves pigment on the carcasses, something consumers prefer not to see. Just like meat chickens, the birds have been genetically altered to grow excessively fast and large—especially in the breast area. As a result, fatal heart attacks among turkeys are so common and economically costly that industry researchers have been asked to study the problem. These turkeys are commonly lame because their spindly legs cannot support their unwieldy bodies. Some are so large and their weight so unevenly distributed that they suffer from what is known as bumble foot, akin to a bedsore on the foot caused by excessive weight and pressure.

The size and shape of the birds have also made it impossible for commercial turkeys to mount and breed naturally. This means that workers at breeding facilities have to masturbate male turkeys, called toms, to collect their semen. Then, in rapid succession, the females are turned upside down and their legs secured by a clamp. The semen is put in straws and inserted into the hen. She's then released from the clamp, making way for the next in line. Not a pleasant process for the bird, nor a job one can take much pride in.

Turkeys suffer from many of the pathologies that afflict broiler chickens, and they experience similar conditions. They also spend most of their lives in crowded grower houses, reaching a slaughter weight of around twenty or thirty pounds at about four months old. Each turkey is allotted roughly three square feet of space in these warehouses, each of which houses thousands of birds. Not surprisingly, the birds cannot perch, run, and forage, never mind forming normal social structures. Because their instincts are frustrated, Ben Franklin's "respectable Bird" is driven to pecking and fighting other turkeys. To lessen injuries, factory-farmed turkeys are debeaked and segments of their toes are cut off, making it easier for catchers and slaughterhouse workers to handle them without being scratched. In some cases, the trauma of these mutilations is fatal; others experience chronic pain as well as difficulty in eating and walking. As in other factory farming processes, workers mutilate the birds in rapid assembly-line fashion, and mistakes are inevitable. I've seen birds so severely debeaked that most of their upper beaks, up to the nostrils, are missing.

Beyond the world of factory farming, it's far too easy for irresponsible individuals to purchase their own flock of turkeys or chickens. Feed stores often post CHICKS AVAILABLE signs, and hard as it may be to believe, it is completely legal to ship many species of domesticated birds, including turkeys, through the mail. In fact, people do it all the time. The birds are packed into boxes, just like clothing or electronics would be. Your order automatically includes more birds than you purchased, since the shipper fully expects some to die in the mail.

A number of the turkeys at the Watkins Glen farm have come from ill-equipped entrepreneurs. People intrigued by the idea of raising turkeys often can't cope with how quickly they grow, how much they eat, and how much waste they produce. The result is badly neglected birds and people desperate to dump the turkeys on someone else. Whisper came from a place like that; she's around two years old and can expect to live another two to three years (a far shorter lifespan than that of a wild turkey). She was one of about eighty turkeys bought by a man who thought he could make good money raising them. He kept the birds in the basement of his house and tried to sell them (unsuccessfully) over the Internet. Turkeys require hands-on care and, like any animal, need to be cleaned up after regularly. It wasn't long before this man's basement was a mess.

Realizing his mistake, he placed an advertisement in the paper, and a local animal rights group called him up and asked him what he was doing. By this time, the man had had enough of being a turkey farmer and offered the group a cut-rate price for the birds. On principle, they refused to pay anything for the birds, and he eventually agreed that the activists could have the turkeys, as long as they came and got them. The local group called Farm Sanctuary to see if we could take in the birds, who were still juveniles, and we agreed. We couldn't house eighty turkeys over the long term, but we could find good homes for most of them. A few, including Whisper, remained at the shelter.

These turkeys hadn't been factory farmed and so still had full beaks and toes. The rescued group included both white and bronze-colored birds, and unusually, the bronzes were the sickly ones. Their legs were splayed and their ligaments irreparably damaged. There simply was no good remedy for them, so we had to euthanize many of them.

The white turkeys, however, were healthy. In a sight that would have made Ben Franklin proud, they flew, admittedly somewhat awkwardly, into trees on the Watkins Glen farm and began to perch, until a whole tree was full of roosting turkeys. Whisper and the other turkeys enjoyed roosting so much that our shelter workers had to climb the trees each evening to bring them into the barn to sleep safely. Ben Franklin might also be happy to know that these turkeys haven't lost their independence. They like to keep an eye on you, and they'll sometimes peck at you or even jump up at you if they're angry. They don't like to be penned in and will put up a fight if cornered.

Other turkeys haven't been so lucky. Chicky and his siblings were dumped in a big box on the front steps of the Watkins Glen farmhouse. They had been rescued from a hatchery that supplies turkey chicks to factory farms and were so tiny they could fit in the palm of your hand. They were sad examples of how erratic the debeaking process on factory farms can be. Fortunately, the debeaking machine had barely clipped Chicky's beak. But others, including Cinnamon, had lost their beak all the way to the nostrils. Some of the poults, as turkey chicks are known, were so badly injured that four died very soon after they arrived at our door. While we treated the survivors' beaks, we set up a nursery where they all recovered nicely.

Nowhere is our collective schizophrenic attitude to turkeys on greater display than at Thanksgiving, where a bird supposed to symbolize failure and stupidity becomes the national symbol of celebration. It's not a celebration of the kind Franklin would have hoped for, and it's on a scale he couldn't have imagined. In 2005, about 256 million turkeys were raised in the United States, one for nearly every American.

Farm Sanctuary celebrates Turkey Day differently. In 1986, we began the Adopt-a-Turkey project, through which people can *save* rather than *serve* turkeys on Thanksgiving Day. Every year, more people participate. Individuals or groups can select a rescued turkey to "adopt" and, for a small donation, we'll send them (or anyone they designate) a photo of "their" turkey, along with a profile, a certificate of adoption, and a set of vegan recipes to help begin a new tradition—a turkey-free Thanksgiving dinner. Many people travel to Watkins Glen and Orland to "turn the tables" and celebrate Thanksgiving by feeding turkeys, not eating them. Instead of being *on* the table, the turkeys get a place *at* the table and feast on traditional Thanksgiving foods such as stuffing, squash, cornbread, mashed potatoes, cranberries, and pumpkin pie. It's a lot of fun for us and our visitors, but we're serious about the message.

The response to the Adopt-a-Turkey program has been remarkable. Over the years, more than a hundred stories about the turkeys at Farm Sanctuary have appeared on network television programs, radio, and websites and in newspapers and magazines, educating millions about alternative ways to express their gratitude. I recall one wonderfully warm November afternoon at our California sanctuary when children held out pumpkin pies, cranberries, and other offerings to the rescued turkeys. They beamed as the birds pecked at the food, then vigorously shook pie filling off their beaks, splattering the delighted children and adults. For us and our visitors, it's a welcome relief from the commercialization that has become a feature of Thanksgiving along with crass ways of "celebrating" such as dropping turkeys out of planes or bowling contests featuring frozen birds.

We've had our share of critics, too—we've been ridiculed by "shock jocks" for sharing the table with our feathered friends rather than eating them. That's a challenge all animal advocacy organizations share. A good portion of the American public would rather not know the grim work that goes into raising their food and don't often think about the animals as individuals. On top of that, we live in an era of cheap stunts, celebrity obsession, reality TV shows, and thirty-second "investigations" on the national news; it can be hard to get the truth out.

For years, actor James Cromwell, a vegetarian and environmentalist who starred as Farmer Hoggett in the movie *Babe*, has participated in our Adopt-a-Turkey program. One year, when asked by a *USA Today* reporter for his thoughts about turkeys' reported low IQs, he responded: "Turkeys have probably been around as long as we have. The only difference is they don't kill each other and they don't pollute the earth. They can't be that dumb."

Ever since 1947, the U.S. president has held an annual Thanksgiving ceremony to "pardon" a turkey. The event, which began as a campaign by the poultry industry to promote turkey consumption during the holiday, always garners substantial publicity. (It also highlights a fact that often goes unquestioned: while wild turkeys may have been consumed at the first Thanksgiving, they were only a small part of the feast. Turkey became a "traditional" part of the Thanksgiving menu only when the poultry industry began promoting the meat as such.)

For years, the pardoned turkeys were sent to a farm in Virginia chosen by the National Turkey Federation, where, it was later discovered, they generally died young. In an effort to remedy the growing public relations disaster, the federation arranged to send the turkeys to Disneyland in 2005, to coincide with the theme park's fiftieth anniversary. My hope is that visitors to the park will connect with the turkeys and learn to appreciate, as I have, how interesting and distinctive these birds are. Perhaps some will join us in our Adopt-a-Turkey celebration, and recognize that the essence of Thanksgiving does not lie in eating a turkey but in gathering together with your family, loved ones, and friends to give thanks and appreciate mercies both big and small. We can do that as easily over mashed yams and stuffed squash or meatless "turkey" entrees as we can over the carcass of a roasted bird.

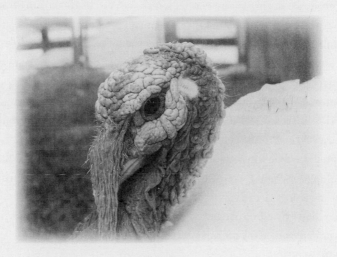

Chicky

PROFILE: CHICKY

In late April 2004, Chicky and nine of his siblings, all of them tiny poults, were rescued from a factory farm hatchery and brought to live at Watkins Glen. Now fully grown and snow white, Chicky weighs thirty-five pounds and has not so much a breast as a double-barreled chest. To ensure he doesn't grow so large that his legs start to suffer from the strain of carrying his own body weight around, Chicky gets half a cup of healthy high-fiber food twice a day. Like all of the male turkeys at Farm Sanctuary, Chicky has a beard, a tuft of long, black, wiry hair in the middle of his chest, and a snood, a flap of skin that hangs over his beak and changes color along with his mood. The snood turns from pale to bright red as more blood flows into it when he's angry or aroused or merely wants to show off. Chicky's generally the first to greet people who stop by the turkey barn. When he's calm, the snood turns bluish white, and at night, when he's sleeping, it's almost completely white.

Chicky is amiable and curious, and he gets on well with everyone on the farm, although, like most males, he becomes aggressive toward other toms during laying season, which in Watkins Glen runs from May to August. Although factory-farmed turkeys such as Chicky are unable to breed, they still try to mount the turkey hens, a potentially risky stunt because of the toms' large size. In addition, turkeys raised for food have been bred to have soft skin, which consumers prefer. Unfortunately for the birds, their soft skin is prone to tears, scrapes, and cuts. We usually keep the male and female turkeys apart to minimize turkey-on-turkey damage. Chicky doesn't know why he's been segregated from the ladies, of course, and you can sometimes see him looking forlornly through the wooden fence that divides him from the hens in the turkey barn. The hens look equally perplexed, but they don't dwell on it, and visitors more often see Chicky and the hens exploring their pastures, scratching in the dirt, and taking naps in the sun.

CHAPTER ELEVEN

Unnatural Disasters

On Monday, August 29, 2005, Hurricane Katrina made landfall on the Gulf Coast of the United States. The hurricane tore through the region, unleashing damaging floods and winds of 125 miles an hour. It devastated New Orleans and the Louisiana and Mississippi coast, left at least seventeen hundred people dead, and forced nearly a quarter of a million people to leave their homes (many of whom have still not been able to return). In addition to the tragic and unprecedented loss of human life, the economic consequences of Katrina totaled nearly $100 billion.

Alongside the millions of people affected by the hurricane were hundreds of thousands of companion animals. Some, left behind when their guardians evacuated, perished when their food and water supplies ran out. Others rode out the storm with their human families, clinging to roofs and porches or taking refuge in attics as the waters rose. When rescue workers arrived, many residents refused to leave without their pets. Reports on these human-animal bonds captivated the country, particularly the story of a little boy who convulsed with sobs when his dog, Snowball, was taken from him before he could board a bus. Calls to allow people to take their dogs and cats with them to emergency shelters grew louder, and officials from the Federal Emergency Management Agency (FEMA) and other agencies eventually relented.

Stories and pictures of cats and dogs in rescue boats became a regular feature of news coverage, as did reunions between families and their pets. But at least one human-animal story didn't capture the Katrina media spotlight and to this day remains relatively unknown. It's the saga of Ginger, Snow White, Cranberry, Grand Master Flash, and the untold

millions of other farmed animals—the vast majority of them chickens—
in Alabama, Florida, Georgia, Louisiana, and Mississippi. They too were
battered and bruised by the storm, and like many of Katrina's victims,
they were left to fend for themselves.

A Chicken in Every Pot

In the 1930s, Tyson began operations in the American South, and as the
poultry industry grew, the South remained its epicenter. Today, poultry
plants in southern states employ about three hundred thousand workers
and supply nearly 90 percent of the nation's broiler chickens. Mississippi
alone accounts for 10 percent of U.S. broiler production. Throughout
the region, the birds are housed in large sheds of, on average, twenty
thousand to twenty-five thousand birds, and raised by contract growers.

Katrina's winds and rain destroyed thousands of these sheds and the
chickens inside. Some drowned in the storm surge, while others were
crushed to death by the collapsing buildings or critically injured by flying debris. Totally dependent on automated feed, water, and ventilation
systems, many other birds died of neglect in the days after Katrina, when
those responsible for their care didn't or couldn't come to their aid. In the
area directly hit by the hurricane, Michael Greger of the Humane Society
of the United States estimated that 100 million broiler chickens were being raised for food. Sanderson Farms is the country's fifth-largest producer
of poultry, with sales of about $1 billion a year. The company reported
that of its nearly two thousand facilities in Mississippi, seventy-two were
destroyed and another eighty-six severely damaged. According to the summer 2005 edition of the *Poultry Health Report*, Sanderson stated that approximately three million head of broiler chickens were destroyed.

In the days after the hurricane, stories of farmed animals abandoned in
Katrina's wake flooded Farm Sanctuary's main office in Watkins Glen. In
Georgia, we learned, a post-Katrina tornado had destroyed thirty chicken
sheds, killing or injuring hundreds of thousands of birds. High winds
in Alabama and Mississippi blew the roofs off dozens of broiler chicken
warehouses, leaving an untold number of birds exposed to severe weather.
In other parts of the Southeast, thousands of chickens drowned.

We also got reports of chickens on the loose. If they lived through the storm, the birds couldn't survive for long without food, water, shelter, or protection from predators. The birds weren't the only animals left to their own devices. We received news of hundreds of cattle in Louisiana trapped in fields, engulfed on all sides by salt water. Other cows on Louisiana's dairy farms faced starvation. Operators couldn't get back to their properties, and shipments of grain for food were halted.

The animal protection community was compelled to respond above and beyond the money, clothes, and food our members and volunteers donated to Katrina's human victims. It was difficult to get the attention of state agricultural authorities or corporate managers for the chickens' plight. The birds' value to the industry is very low, and our society in general doesn't value them much higher. In any case, the chickens in the hurricane zone were property and, like some of the homes and possessions lost to Katrina, they were insured. This meant the corporate owners could collect on their damaged or destroyed "goods."

Most of the region's poultry processing plants stayed idle in the days following Katrina, as they lacked a steady supply of chickens or workers. According to figures from Mississippi's agriculture department, six million chickens were killed when the poultry sheds were destroyed. The industry's priority was cleaning up the chickens, dead or alive, not rescuing them. Yet, even if the owners had wanted to do something else, the scale of chicken production in the region is so enormous that it's nearly impossible to protect the birds or relocate them when something goes wrong. How could a million chickens be evacuated, let alone tens of millions of animals? Not that animal agriculture considered developing a contingency plan: it was cheaper to do cleanup and collect on the insurance.

The Humane Society of the United States, Animal Place (a sanctuary in California), and Farm Sanctuary together sent a team of rescuers to the region. The team, which was joined by other groups and individual activists, reported seeing mass graves where dead and dying birds had been dumped. Fields were littered with dead chickens, and others ran helplessly about. As much as the flooded roads allowed them to, the team went farm to farm in Mississippi in search of live chickens in the sheds, outside their shattered remains, and in the vast open graves.

Many of the contract growers refused the team's pleas to rescue the chickens. Because the growers didn't own the birds, they were fearful of what would happen if they gave away the inventory. Meanwhile, hundreds of thousands of dead and live birds were being bulldozed, along with the remains of the damaged broiler sheds, into freshly dug holes. This had become an accepted way of disposing of the "debris" left by the hurricane. "We saw a massive open grave containing thousands of dead chickens crawling with maggots," Kate Walker, a Farm Sanctuary staffer and team member, reported. "Shockingly, twenty-one birds were still alive, huddled in the corner of the pit."

The team did find one grower with a different attitude. One of his sheds had been destroyed and others damaged. He was under contract to an integrator, whose managers had told him to move the surviving chickens into a shed that was still standing. But it didn't feel right to him to crowd more birds into a shed that, in line with industry standards, was already crammed full of birds. After some discussion, he agreed to let the animal rescuers have the birds. He acted in the chickens' best interests, but his decision could have gotten him into legal trouble with the integrator, one of the leading agribusiness corporations. This really does characterize the heartlessness of industrial farming. Animals are first and foremost live "stock," like commodities traded on Wall Street.

The team also visited facilities from which broilers had escaped or been thrown by Katrina's force. The chickens were scattered everywhere, dazed and dehydrated. A few found shelter and perhaps some food under berry bushes. When the rescuers got to them, the birds' feathers were stained with berry juice, a testament of sorts to their will to survive. Appropriately, the shelter staff later named one of these hens Cranberry. When the team found animals hopelessly suffering, they made the difficult decision to put them out of their misery.

The team got as many live chickens out of Mississippi as they could. All in all, they saved about eleven hundred, of which around seven hundred made the journey north to Watkins Glen. Animal Place took a hundred and the Black Beauty Ranch, a Texas animal shelter, took three hundred. The chickens had probably hatched in early August and were about two to three weeks away from slaughter. I'm proud of what the rescue team did and the role Farm Sanctuary played. But more than six million farmed animals, mostly chickens, had lost their lives in Katrina's path. Those we saved were a straw in a mountain of hay. To me, though, they are all individuals who deserve protection, care, kindness, and a decent life.

When the Katrina chickens first arrived at Farm Sanctuary, the shelter staff worked long hours taking care of them. The birds were suffering from a combination of the effects of the hurricane and genetic manipulation. Many had difficulty walking because they were so heavy. Lack of proper feed had left their bones weak and prone to break. Many of the hens and roosters also had broken toes, had severe gangrene in their feet, and suffered from dehydration and a lack of nutrition. One bird's eye was swollen shut from trauma to the head, while another had a large head wound.

Shelter staff, working around the clock, administered IV fluids, painkillers, and steroids and kept the birds on heating pads to stabilize them in our hospital area. The first night they were at the shelter, a late summer thunderstorm crashed through the area. Twelve of the birds died then from flip-over syndrome, and over the next few months, forty more died the same way. We've learned a lot by working with the Katrina birds. When they first arrived, the hens had a very strong urge to eat, the result of selective breeding that fueled their fast growth. They tried eating everything they could peck at.

At about a year old—ten months beyond their slaughter age—the Katrina hens weighed around ten pounds and the roosters around fifteen pounds. That's twice and three times their respective slaughter weights. They can hardly walk, let alone run or fly. To extend their lives and help with their mobility, we've put them on a high-fiber diet and restricted portion sizes. They get half a cup of feed in the morning each (specially mixed pellets with vitamins) and the same thing at night—the most nutrition on the least calories possible. It's a delicate balance, to provide good nutrition while limiting weight gain. In commercial chicken sheds, they'd be on a concentrated fast-growth diet, plus antibiotics, and have access to food around the clock. No wonder they're prone to heart attacks.

The chickens have proved intriguing in other ways. Some of the shelter staff call them the "X-Files" birds because their eggs have double yolks. As producers have engineered bigger and faster-growing birds, they have increased certain behavioral and physical traits. Perhaps double-yolk eggs are one. The eggs laid by Katrina hens are much larger than the ones the rescued battery hens lay. But they also have soft shells, are often misshapen, and vary in color. The birds' unwieldy bodies are taxed just to function on a daily basis, and laying fully formed eggs is sometimes beyond them.

We work hard to provide all our birds with proper nutrition, including their calcium intake. This includes hard-boiling the eggs the hens lay and adding them to the chickens' feed, which helps replenish their calcium. After being rescued, broiler birds will typically live only one or two years. They just aren't built for longevity, and unfortunately, there's nothing we can do to change that.

We have also found that some of the Katrina roosters are *extremely* aggressive with the hens, each other, some of the male Farm Sanctuary turkeys, and even the staff. When fully grown, the largest male roosters can weigh about twenty pounds. In addition to their large legs, they have large feet and spurs, a stiff spiny claw on the back that they use to fight with or express dominance. The roosters' spur strikes can tear into all kinds of skin (bird and human) and have done so. When they were young they were very sweet, but as they matured, a number changed dramatically.

Some of the Katrina roosters and a few hens have been injured in fights and, even more alarmingly, rapes committed by other Katrina roosters, particularly the largest ones. As they try to mount hens and even smaller roosters, the larger males tear up the other birds' feathers and skin, which is why we won't put any hen with an aggressive rooster. Twenty of the Katrina hens now live in a flock with Pedro, a small reddish-colored rooster who was rescued with Marmalade and others following a cruelty investigation at a farm in Prattsburgh, New York. Pedro is barely half the size of the hens, but they're a good match—everyone's happy. We've had to move the male roosters who've been attacked into a separate pasture, so they can regroup and regain their confidence.

In the past, we have had roosters scuffle at Farm Sanctuary, but nothing like this. When we do health checks on the Katrina roosters or give them medications, the staff wears Kevlar gloves up to their elbows to protect their arms from spurs and beaks. The roosters also exhibit behaviors we've never seen before. For instance, some tried to eat one another's feces when they were put on restricted diets after a necessary surgery. That is not normal bird behavior.

Some of what we see in the roosters might be due to excess testosterone (in commercial production the roosters don't live long enough to reach sexual maturity). Their aberrant behaviors are by-products of the genetic engineering practiced by the industry—and it's disturbing, to say the least. Temple Grandin describes being at a chicken facility and seeing a bloodied hen, dead on the floor. The farmer, unfazed, told her a rooster had killed the hen. Grandin wrote, "I knew that couldn't be right. If roosters killed hens in nature, there wouldn't be any chickens." The farmer said that half of his roosters were what she calls "rapist-murderers." The rooster's aggression, Grandin explains, was an unintended side effect of what's called "single trait breeding." The goal is fast growth and heavy muscles to increase the amount of meat on each bird. The result, Grandin writes, is "warped evolution." What had been lost in at least half of the roosters was the rooster courtship program.

Most roosters do a dance of sorts before they try to mate with a hen. When the hen sees the dance, she moves her body into a position that allows the rooster to mount her easily. But, as Grandin points out, if the hen doesn't see the dance, she doesn't crouch down. So when the rooster mounts anyway, by force, he injures the hen, often fatally. The farmers and breeders didn't recognize that they'd created monsters. "As the roosters got more and more aggressive," Grandin notes, "the humans unconsciously adjusted their perceptions of how a normal rooster should act." "Rapist roosters" have become an accepted part of the production process, a cost of doing business that has been largely hidden on factory farms. But not at Farm Sanctuary.

Since they arrived, we have spent thousands of dollars on veterinary care for the Katrina birds, much more than we ever anticipated. But Farm Sanctuary has never, even in the early days, denied an animal needed care or medicines because of cost. We're thankful we've received great support from our members, which allows us to look after the animals, and for which I will always be grateful. Several hundred of the Katrina chickens were eventually adopted out to good homes.

The qualities that make hens and roosters chickens have no market value, so "animal science" gives no thought to maintaining them. As in the case of the Katrina birds, their behaviors have become so disordered that they're practically pathological. Animal science has made it very hard for these chickens to live full lives without physical difficulty or pain. But as you can see at Farm Sanctuary every day, it has not eliminated their desires or abilities to bathe in the dust, preen, establish a pecking order, and for some, to rule the roost.

Nature's Fury

Hurricane Katrina wasn't the first weather-related emergency to propel Farm Sanctuary into high gear. On September 20, 2000, tornadoes sped through Croton, Ohio, destroying homes, toppling trees, and ripping apart twelve buildings belonging to Buckeye Egg Farm. Inside the buildings were over a million birds, caged in vast rows and stacked three tiers high. The winds tore off the shed roofs, revealing a nightmarish scene very few people ever see. Everywhere you looked were warped and mangled cages stuffed with chickens. Many had been suffocated or crushed to death; others were critically injured. Some of the cages had either partially or wholly broken open, leaving birds dangling or flapping around desperately. The majority of hens, however, remained trapped without access to food or water, since most of the troughs and feeders in front of the cages had been disconnected or twisted by the winds out of the birds' reach.

When Farm Sanctuary heard about the tornado and its aftermath, we joined up with Jason Tracy and Cayce Mell, who at the time ran OohMahNee Sanctuary in Pennsylvania. We wanted to send a team to rescue as many birds as we could. But first we had to plead with Buckeye's owners by fax and phone to be granted permission to do so. After days of going back and forth, animal advocates were allowed to join the company's "rescue" team, which consisted of half a dozen men who grabbed birds by their legs in big bunches and threw them onto a truck. The truck then deposited the birds into a large dumpster, which was covered with a tarpaulin. The workers pumped carbon dioxide into the closed space for five minutes, then dumped more birds on top; those who had survived the gas were then crushed or suffocated to death by the next truckload. Half a million birds were disposed of this way—and eventually piled into pits with refuse and unusable machinery.

Farm Sanctuary and OohMahNee's staff and volunteers, along with animal advocates in Ohio, weren't interested in treating the chickens as debris. Instead, they gathered the birds in their arms (a humane practice that was emulated by some members of the Buckeye team), and over the next twelve days they collected about three thousand hens. We called on Farm Sanctuary's entire Farm Animal Adoption Network to adopt the chickens, and our friends and supporters came through. Eventually, we took a thousand to Watkins Glen. The rescued birds who survived the carnage at Buckeye suffered many reproductive and other illnesses due to the intense strain put on their bodies by the production of so many eggs. Still, Tofutti Cutie, Taboo, Milky Way, and others were able to enjoy the rest of their lives with a degree of comfort denied to their fellow Buckeye layer hens.

Emerging Ailments

When a catastrophic event strikes a factory farm, the farmed animals aren't the only victims. It's just about impossible to control what happens to the pathogens that thrive on factory farms. When Hurricane Floyd struck North Carolina in 1999, for instance, torrential rain and flooding caused hog factory manure lagoons to overflow their banks and pollute the surrounding countryside with the waste. Four years before that, lagoons of hog manure had burst, on that occasion contaminating drinking water and killing vast numbers of fish in nearby rivers.

For as long as humans have been on this planet, viruses and bacteria have been with us. We have evolved and developed resistance and tolerance to most of them. But we are now at the point where our farming system has created vast monocultures (genetically similar strains) of animals and housed them in conditions where diseases can easily spread. Thanks to the industry's excessive and irresponsible use of antibiotics in farmed animals, we are creating the ideal environment for terrible sicknesses to develop.

Concerned that antibiotic resistance is a "big problem and growing," Linda Tollefson, director of surveillance and compliance at the U.S. Food and Drug Administration's Center for Veterinary Medicine, explains, "You're dealing with living microbes that have shown an incredible ability to accommodate antibiotics and come out winning. We have no idea what they are going to do next. Our fear is that we're seeing the tip of the iceberg."

"Antibiotic use really pushes the evolutionary process to favor organisms that are resistant," says Stuart Levy, M.D., director of the Center for Adaptation Genetics and Drug Resistance at Tufts University School of Medicine. "Any individuals in the bacterial population that is being targeted that happen to have genes that give them resistance to the antibiotic will survive and multiply." Dr. Theresa Smith of the U.S. Centers for Disease Control and Prevention goes so far as saying that the evolution of virulent bacterial resistance "threatens to return us to the era before the development of antibiotics."

Of pressing concern currently is the possible spread of avian influenza, or bird flu, which has already been found in many countries in Africa, Asia, and Europe. At Farm Sanctuary we are in the process of putting together a plan for how to deal with highly pathogenic avian flu if and when it comes to North America.

Avian influenza has mutated to become transmissible from one person to another before, most virulently between 1918 and 1920. Millions of people died worldwide, and if it breaks out again on a mass scale, it could be even more serious. There are more of us in existence who might catch and spread the disease, and we're better connected to each other than ever before with global trade and international travel at an all-time high. Moreover, today there are vast numbers of farm animals, especially birds, who are weak, genetically similar, and unable to fend off illnesses.

Recent speculation suggesting that wild birds can transport and transmit bird flu as they migrate has led some industry experts to advocate that all domesticated birds be moved indoors. They argue that keeping captive birds completely separated from wild birds will minimize spread of the flu. Agribusiness especially likes to point the finger of blame at unfettered animals and rural people in poor countries who keep chickens in their backyard. They didn't have the means to defend themselves from allegations that their flocks are the cause of a disease that might spread to U.S. domestic poultry.

Some animal health experts, however, dispute this hypothesis. They suggest that the opposite could be true. Hon Ip, a virologist with the U.S. Geological Survey's National Wildlife Health Center, believes that virulent strains of bird flu most likely evolved in *domesticated* poultry. Factory-farmed birds who live short lives and are housed together in confined spaces with thousands of others provide the ideal environment for such resilient pathogens to develop. Dr. Michael Greger in his book *Bird Flu: A Virus of Our Own Hatching*, a comprehensive study of the causes of avian influenza, concluded that the risk of a pandemic outbreak of a strain of the flu that could spread from humans to other humans is greatly enhanced by the industrial confinement methods used to raise food animals.

Even some in the industry are beginning to question the assumption that wild birds are the main culprits in the spread of this disease. According to Meatingplace.com, a meat industry news source, "Scientists have been unable to link the spread of bird flu to migratory patterns, suggesting thousands of wild birds that have died are not primary transmitters of the virus and that shipments of domestic poultry pose a far greater threat." The article also notes that infected poultry litter from commercial farms may play a role in spreading the disease.

Although the current and particularly virulent strain of avian flu, H5N1, has only recently come to the public's attention, variants of bird flu have been detected in commercial poultry flocks in the United States for years. In some cases, infected birds have been killed to prevent the spread of these diseases. But other infected birds have entered the human food supply. In 2000, after Queenie the cow's escape from a halal slaughterhouse in the New York City borough of Queens, people living nearby pressured city officials to close down the facility. After investigating the neighbors' complaints, they found numerous violations and ordered the slaughterhouse closed. Farm Sanctuary offered to take in the remaining animals, including 150 terrified chickens found in dozens of crowded cages stacked three and four high. Live birds were mixed in with dead ones, the wire cages were caked with excrement, and there was no water or food in sight. (City officials later confirmed that the birds had been left without food or water for days.) We transported the birds to Watkins Glen.

In a bizarre twist, we learned that it is illegal to remove birds from slaughterhouses because of concerns about spreading disease, though it's perfectly legal to kill poultry infected with strains of avian influenza for use in human food. The USDA required us to run tests for avian flu, though the birds would have been slaughtered and sold for food without such testing. The tests came back positive, and we had to house these birds in their own area separate from all the other animals. Farm Sanctuary had been passed the buck once again.

With avian influenza infecting birds throughout the world, millions, perhaps hundreds of millions, are being culled. A number of people are now confirmed to have died from avian flu in several countries, and, as of this writing, there is evidence that human-to-human transmission of the virus may have occurred in at least one case. The potential for devastation from the spread of the disease is very real. But while we speculate about bird flu, the fact remains that other pathogens commonly found in U.S. poultry, such as salmonella and campylobacter, quietly continue to kill many people in the United States each year.

Out of Sight, Out of Mind

In a recent report, the USDA estimated that Hurricane Katrina resulted in $30 million worth of "livestock losses." Ironically, before Katrina hit, the National Chicken Council had declared September 2005 "National Chicken Month" to boost sales of its products. A week after the hurricane, the USDA *Broiler Market News Report* described the situation for broilers and fryers in the South this way: "In production areas, live supplies were moderate at mixed, but mostly desirable weights." It was back to business as usual.

Albert Einstein once said, "We can't solve problems by using the same kind of thinking we used when we created them." Katrina revealed the deep economic and racial divides that still exist in the United States and that too often go unacknowledged and unaddressed. Of course, the storm also showed Americans volunteering, taking in the displaced, and working together to help those affected. This caring spirit was on display not just for humans but for the animals who live with us. Now, I'm not naive enough to believe that untold millions of animals could all be rescued by a few passionate, hardworking people, and, obviously, drastic events call for drastic measures. But Katrina uncovered how many pressing issues mainstream American society has deliberately pushed to the margins of consciousness. It also demonstrated how woefully unprepared this country is for catastrophic events.

As the global climate changes, these events will only grow more intense and frequent, leading to even greater human and animal displacement and larger economic losses. Too often ignored in this is the way our food choices affect the planet. Our appetite for meat is actually fueling global warming and other major environmental problems. According to a 2006 report from the United Nations Food and Agriculture Organization entitled *Livestock's Long Shadow*, animal farming is responsible for 18 percent of global greenhouse gas emissions, a larger share than that contributed by transportation. "Livestock are one of the most significant contributors to today's most serious environmental problems," said Henning Steinfeld, the report's senior author. "Urgent action is required to remedy the situation." The livestock industry is also competing for land, water, and other natural resources that are already scarce in many parts of the world.

What does it say about our society that so many of the victims of Katrina were virtually invisible to us after the storm hit? Or that the misery and death of millions of animals went largely unnoticed, rating a shrug of indifference even from the farmers charged with their care? *Half a billion* living creatures, *half a billion* painful deaths, were all written off as just another "economic loss" before everyone got back to business.

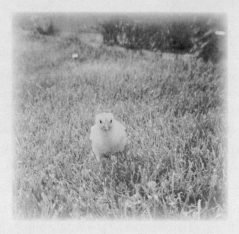

Mayfly

PROFILE: MAYFLY

Mayfly is one of the most popular roosters at Farm Sanctuary, friendly to our human visitors and caring toward his twenty or so layer hen companions, all of whom were rescued from the Buckeye Egg Farm in Ohio in 2000. At five or six years old, these "old ladies" like to spend time in the shade and under the blackberry bushes with Mayfly. Mayfly has been at the Watkins Glen shelter since he was just a day old, which may account for his ease with staff and visitors. He lets us pick him up and give him a hug every now and then. Mayfly was part of a school hatching project. A group of eggs were incubated and broken open (one each day), to show students how chicks develop inside the shell.

One day, the teacher had had enough. She didn't much like what the project entailed, and decided to let the final two chicks hatch on their own. One was Mayfly. Soon afterward, though, the chicks got wet—bad news for any newborn chick. They can't tolerate water at that age; they can get sick and even die. Mother hens sit on their chicks and protect them, and if it rains, they'll spread their wings to keep the water from reaching the babies. But these chicks didn't have a mother hen around.

Luckily, one of the mothers of a child in the class brought the wet chicks to us, very upset, and begged us to help them. We agreed to take them in, and through veterinary care and attention, Mayfly survived. Sadly, the other chick didn't. Mayfly has grown into a genial and responsible rooster. In fact, he's one of the best roosters on the farm at protecting his hens, which is any rooster's primary job. Animal experts have documented twenty-two recognizable and distinct vocalizations in roosters. One call encourages all the hens to move. Another alerts them to the fact that there's food to be eaten. And another alerts the hens to danger from the sky. When there's a hawk flying over the farm, Mayfly makes a high-pitched noise that sets off a race among the hens to the barn. Mayfly then runs around the yard making sure everyone is all right. Only when he's satisfied his charges have reached safety does he go into the barn himself.

PART THREE

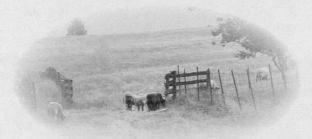

ON THEIR
BEHALF—
AND OURS

CHAPTER TWELVE

In the Eyes of the Law

In the years since Farm Sanctuary's founding, our work has involved both rescuing abused or abandoned farm animals and "going upstream," working to change conditions institutionally and systemically. To meet our goals we need to reach out to the public and the business community to help support the enactment and enforcement of laws and policies to protect farm animals. Our first journey upstream was with the no-downer campaign that began at Lancaster Stockyards. Since then, we have been involved in a number of campaigns to change laws and policies—some successful, others still in progress. In this chapter, I want to share some recent examples of this work, and to say again why it's so important.

Laws have always served to codify a society's values. They reflect our character and, at times, our aspirations. With new awareness, our worldview changes and evolves, and so do our laws. At one time, slavery and child labor were common and assumed to be normal and economically essential practices. But over time they came to be widely understood as unjust and unacceptable. We've also enacted animal protection laws that acknowledge that we are responsible for treating other animals with kindness and respect.

As far back as 1641, the Massachusetts Bay colony enacted "The Body of Liberties," which included a provision that read, "No man shall exercise any Tiranny or Cruelty towards any brute Creature which are usually kept for man's use." However, in the case of animals raised for food, current laws are out of sync with our societal values. As modern factory farming developed its hyperefficient methods, focusing entirely on production and all but ignoring animal welfare, animal cruelty laws were amended to exclude farm animals. With each new efficiency-promoting idea the question within the industry was always whether something *could* be done and not whether it *should* be done at all.

Millions of people are buying meat and other animal products from a system that is so repugnant that even industry insiders are concerned that factory farming conditions are inhumane. Numerous public opinion surveys show a vast majority of people in the United States and around the globe are uneasy with industrialized animal farming. It doesn't sit well on our conscience, leaving exactly two options: we can live in denial, looking the other way, or we can find it in ourselves to confront the cruelty and do something about it.

When I speak with lawmakers and urge them to support legislation prohibiting the cruel treatment of farm animals, I'm often told that you cannot legislate morality. But that is exactly what laws do: they uphold societal values and ethics. They assert standards of decency and define the boundary between right and wrong, responsible and irresponsible, acceptable and unacceptable.

In turning away from the abuses of factory farming, we have allowed the industry to establish positions of influence within the government and other institutions. It's time to face industrial agribusiness, whose blindness to the suffering of animals is almost equaled by their indifference to the well-being of the public. Our health, the appropriation of scarce planetary resources, food security, and how we treat other animals cannot be left to corporations and the government alone. The character of our country is at issue here. We need to communicate with those we have elected to work for the common good, and make sure that unsustainable and inhumane factory farms do not jeopardize our future.

Our current laws permit routine abuse on factory farms and prevent those responsible from being held accountable. I spend more and more of my time these days working to change laws or encourage policies to prevent this cruelty. Laws, however, are only as good as their enforcement, which is why we're also trying to ensure that laws on the books are more than just words on a page. That is why education is crucial—not only of legislators and law enforcement agents but of the public at large. We need a better-informed citizenry to participate in the process and help change the status quo, and that's where you come in.

More times than I can say, I have asked myself how we as a society could collectively fail to provide the vast majority of animals under our care with even the most basic humane protection. How could we come to accept that the massive institutional cruelty at the center of factory farming is normal? How did it all come to pass?

In part, at least, the answer is ignorance. Most people don't realize that legal protections for farmed animals in the United States are virtually nonexistent. For its part, the farmed animal industry has, according to attorneys Mariann Sullivan and David Wolfson, performed "an extraordinary legal sleight of hand. It has made farmed animals disappear from the law." This has happened even though, "[f]rom a statistician's point of view, since farmed animals represent 98 percent of all animals with whom humans interact in the United States, all animals are farmed animals; the number that are not is statistically insignificant."

Farm animals are specifically excluded from the federal Animal Welfare Act, which regulates the treatment of animals in other industries. But two other federal laws should pertain to farm animals. One, known as the twenty-eight-hour law, says that farm animals cannot be transported more than twenty-eight hours without being rested. The law, which was written in 1872, when trains were the primary means of transport, had been interpreted to apply only to trains, not trucks, the primary method of transportation today. In 2006, the USDA responded to a petition brought by humane groups and agreed that the twenty-eight-hour law *does* apply to farm animals shipped by truck. But this interpretation hasn't changed much on the ground. The twenty-eight-hour law is still not being enforced.

Ironically, or perhaps fittingly, the most pertinent law protecting farm animals is the Humane Methods of Slaughter Act, which requires, in theory anyway, that animals be rendered insensible to pain prior to being bled to death. But it has been interpreted to exclude poultry, and even in the case of mammals it has not been properly enforced. Numerous investigations continue to document persistent violations of the act in the nation's slaughterhouses.

While nations in Europe have explicitly recognized all animals, including farm animals, as sentient beings who deserve to be treated with respect, laws in the United States fail to do so and exclude farm animals.

This allows them to be treated as the industry sees fit, as mere product, akin to the cars or any other consumer goods that roll off an assembly line. And while most states have anti-cruelty statutes that prohibit animal abuse, agribusiness, wanting to avoid any risk of prosecution, has, since the 1980s, set out to change humane laws. And so, state by state, the industry has worked to exclude customary farming practices from those laws, and thereby deny farm animals basic protection. In most cases, agribusiness has succeeded.

The result is that conduct that would be considered cruelty to a dog or a cat—denial of food, water, shelter, and veterinary care, as well as being chained or confined in cages or crates in conditions that cause both physical and psychological disorders—is often lawful and, alarmingly, standard practice in the treatment of billions of farm animals in the United States. Fearful of appearing to be "against" farming, state lawmakers have, as Sullivan and Wolfson write, "endowed the farmed-animal industry with complete authority to define what is, and what is not, cruelty to the animals in their care." In practice, this means that the farmed-animal industry has "persuaded the majority of state legislatures to amend their criminal anticruelty statutes to exempt all 'accepted,' 'common,' 'customary,' or 'normal' farming practices." Any activity, no matter how cruel, may be considered legal as long as the industry adopted it as "normal."

In a majority of states in this country, farming exemptions have been enacted into laws that put no limits on how animals are treated on the farm as long as what is done to them is "customary." This means that if the industry wants to institute a new method of raising farmed animals and does so on a widespread basis, judges, prosecutors, or the local SPCA can't take any action—even if the result is massive suffering. The effect is to put billions of animals beyond the reach of the law; it's as if they don't even exist. According such sweeping power to an industry to dictate laws is unprecedented in this country. "It is difficult to imagine another nongovernmental group possessing such influence over criminal legal definition," as Sullivan and Wolfson conclude.

So you see how incredibly difficult it is to bring charges against factory farms, even when apparently blatant examples of outrageous cruelty have been documented with video footage, photos, and eyewitness testimony.

The defense simply argues that the practices are accepted or normal and so legally protected. Case dismissed. But the inconsistencies in the law are absurd. An animal used for meat, milk, or eggs has virtually no protections, but if the same animal was kept as somebody's companion, he or she would have protection under existing laws. Our subjective intentions regarding animals versus the objective cruelty they're exposed to determines whether or not they are provided any humane protection.

As if the legal protections for their industry's practices weren't weak enough, agribusiness also has lobbied successfully for legislation that provides it with tax breaks and government subsidies, along with exemptions from environmental, labor, and antitrust laws. Over the years, industry lobbyists have consistently thwarted legislative proposals to protect animals, workers, consumers, and the environment, even as agribusiness wraps itself in the myth of protecting the family farm. Even the names of some of these groups, such as Farmers for Clean Air and Water, cleverly obscure the reality of agribusiness attempting to avoid any regulation of its practices, including the safe disposal of toxic manure from factory farms. Perhaps no other American industry has ever enjoyed the same level of protection and privilege as modern agribusiness. Perhaps none has had so many state and federal officials ready to do its bidding. History has shown that entities that grow to such power and dominance usually fall by their own cruel and corrupt excesses, which may yet be the fate of factory farming.

Property or "Persons"

One of the defining problems of pursuing farmed animal abuse charges is that, under the law, animals are considered property, like a tractor or a plow. The battle over what or who is considered property and who deserves consideration has been fought over and over again in the history of this country. The founders enshrined the right of protest and freedom of speech in the U.S. Constitution and the Bill of Rights, even as they denied some individuals freedom, property, or the ability to vote. And from that point forward there's been a struggle between those who claim the law should protect the status quo and those—such as abolitionists, suffragists, and civil rights activists—who argue that certain laws are unjust and so need to change. I agree with the Reverend Dr. Martin Luther King Jr. in his belief that "the arc of the moral universe is long, but it bends toward justice."

A noted writer in *The Washington Post* recently described the cause of compassion for farm animals as "the moral calling of our time." Like other struggles before it, the animal protection movement seeks to free oppressed individuals from cruelty and injustice. We see animals as flesh-and-blood beings with their own interests and needs, rather than property to be abused and exploited as the legal owner deems suitable. We see the animals' vulnerability and their degradation at the hands of cruel men or cruel systems. We also see how human beings degrade themselves through such acts of cruelty.

This cause does not seek to provide animals with the same rights that oppressed people have fought for over centuries. That's a false caricature of our movement, promoted by industries that profit from animal suffering. In reality, the animal protection cause simply asks that animals not be treated like things but respected as creatures with inherent rights. It also maintains that we have an ethical responsibility not to abuse them. Asserting the rights of animals to be protected from human cruelty is just the affirmative version of the timeless principle that it is wrong to treat them cruelly.

As we discover how complex animals of all kinds are—how rich their inner lives, how sophisticated their communication, and how carefully structured their social networks—it becomes difficult to ignore their claims on us. We know, as a scientific matter, much more about other animals than did our ancestors. With this knowledge comes a clearer responsibility, but also a greater opportunity. By extending the reach of human compassion we make the world a better place for animals and for ourselves.

An 1886 Supreme Court decision (*Santa Clara County v. Southern Pacific Railroad Company*) defined corporations as persons with many of the same legal rights and protections as individuals. But unlike corporations or, of course, human beings, animals do not have what's known as legal standing. This makes going to court to protect them, and Farm Sanctuary's work, even harder. As a general matter, the law permits an injured party to bring an action. When farm animals are abused, it is *they* who are injured and not Farm Sanctuary. In spite of this general rule, which overlooks the general public interest in preventing cruel and unjust conduct, we have worked to gain legal standing to defend farm animals from abuse, and on a few occasions we have been authorized to bring suit.

One of our successes, in terms of gaining standing, came after we filed suit against the California Department of Food and Agriculture for its regulations that exempted the ritual slaughter of poultry from the humane slaughter law (California has a unique state law that applies to poultry). The department asserted that Farm Sanctuary was not affected by the law and so did not have the standing to sue. It argued that the case should be dismissed without discussing the merits. But the appellate court thought otherwise and ruled that Farm Sanctuary should have standing. It concluded:

> We realize that Farm Sanctuary and its members might not face any hardship if we decline to reach the merits of the case. The HSL [Humane Slaughter Law] was enacted for the benefit of animals. If the ritualistic slaughter regulation is invalid, it will result in an unlawful injury to poultry, not humans. In essence, the affected animals in this case are the real parties in interest. In these unique circumstances, we should focus on the potential harm to the beneficiaries of the statute. . . . Further, as a practical matter, Farm Sanctuary should be allowed to challenge the ritualistic slaughter regulation.

The court's decision also said: "[U]nless an organization like Farm Sanctuary is permitted to challenge the department's rulemaking authority, the ritualistic slaughter regulation will be immune from judicial review." In the view of Sheldon Eisenberg, one of Farm Sanctuary's lawyers, the language of the decision is a "significant advance in the extremely technical law of 'standing,'" based on a "commonsense" response to real-world considerations. Looking to the future, the court's ruling could, according to Eisenberg, have a major impact if it's applied in other standing contexts and "hopefully may lead to further eroding some of the legal barriers that exist to obtaining justice for animals."

Of course, the point the appellate court made in its decision applies equally to all such cases: to deny the right of Farm Sanctuary or others to bring challenges on behalf of cruelly treated animals, and on behalf of the public interest in preventing cruelty, is in effect to remove the entire issue from the purview of any court. In other words, industry would never have to answer for alleged violations of the law.

Sometimes we're the ones being charged, when, incredibly, our efforts to treat farm animals humanely are met with criminal prosecution. In late 2002, Susie Coston, our shelter director, responded to a cruelty call about a sheep farm a few miles down the road from our Watkins Glen shelter. When there was no response to her knocks on the farmhouse door, she searched the grounds for someone to talk to—but no one was around. Through an open door of the barn, Susie saw a small lamb whose back legs were paralyzed and whose eyes were crusted shut.

The other sheep crowded together in the barn were trampling the lamb, and Susie naturally removed him from the danger. She washed the crust from his eyes, cleaned his feces-soaked wool, and took him in for veterinary care. The vet told Susie that the lamb had a broken back along with a host of other problems and that there was no hope of recovery. Sadly, euthanizing him was the decision that made the most sense. The lamb had clearly not received appropriate care and attention, and we believed the farmer should be prosecuted for animal cruelty. Instead, to our amazement, Susie was charged—with felony burglary.

Animal advocates across the United States came to her defense. The office of the district attorney (DA) received thousands of calls and letters urging that the farmer and not Susie be charged. "If you saw a child drowning in a pool in a neighbor's yard, would you trespass to save the child?" I asked the DA. "Or, would you give the no-trespassing law higher priority?" The DA didn't have a strong case and Susie had no prior criminal record, and he eventually reduced the charge to criminal trespass, a misdemeanor. In a plea bargain, Susie was required to perform a hundred hours of community service, write a letter of apology to the farmer, and, adding insult to injury, pay restitution of $200, which included the value of the lamb. But even that wasn't enough for the New York State Farm Bureau. They pressured the DA, who called me into his office and put me on notice that if anything like this happened again, "somebody would go to jail."

Over the years all kinds of rescued animals have been anonymously left at Farm Sanctuary's door. The owner, and abuser, of these animals might consider them stolen property that we should rightfully return. But if the animal is sick and suffering, don't we have a higher moral obligation to provide him or her with the necessary care the owner didn't see fit to provide? A mere 150 years ago the Underground Railroad sheltered human beings in much the same way—slaves who under the law were considered property were hidden from their owners for fear they would be harmed, or worse, if they were returned. The Underground Railroad and some of its best-known conductors, including Harriet Tubman, were active in the region surrounding Watkins Glen (Tubman's preserved house is in Auburn, New York, about sixty miles away), and to my thinking, we follow in their footsteps.

Laws and Labels

To change the law, we need to work hand in hand with legislators—but that's not to say it's easy. In the United States, state and federal legislative bodies are typically organized into committees that focus on particular issues, such as international affairs, banking, defense, and agriculture. Agriculture committees include lawmakers who represent agricultural districts, and they tend to promote the interests of their constituents, often to the detriment of the public good. I've seen people deliver passionate, compelling testimony before state agriculture committees, only to be met with impassive and uninterested stares, or even hostility, from committee members. The symbiotic relationship between government and agribusiness has certainly influenced their cavalier attitudes.

Agribusiness, however, is getting nervous, as awareness of animal suffering in factory farms has spread. A 2008 Gallup poll found that nearly two-thirds of Americans "support passing strict laws concerning the treatment of farm animals." A number of other polls conducted in recent years by Zogby and others consistently find that a strong majority of Americans consider industrial farming practices to be cruel and unacceptable. And in a 2004 survey of U.S. veterinarians, 80 percent of the respondents expressed their opinion that veal crates, gestation crates, and battery cages were objectionable.

As a result, some change is afoot. For instance, with the supply of eggs exceeding demand, the egg industry is now planning to provide layer hens with more space. The allotment will increase from approximately 48 square inches per bird to 67 inches per bird. While this is a step in the right direction, it remains grossly inadequate. A single bird needs around 303 square inches, just to flap her wings.

Still, for the most part the industry goes on the offensive to discourage reform, with tactics ranging from the frightening to the absurd. Agribusiness advisers have warned farmers that reading books such as *Bambi* or *Charlotte's Web* to children or allowing them to see a film such as *Babe* can "infect" them with the "animal rights virus." Far more disturbing are the sustained efforts of men such as former Texas representative Charles Stenholm, who spent much of the 1990s blocking passage of the Downed Animal Protection Act. He along with others in Congress have worked to make sure that well-meaning people who advocate for animals are marginalized, if not criminalized.

In 1992, a decade before the terrorist attacks of September 11, 2001, Stenholm co-sponsored the Animal Enterprise Protection Act, which led to various animal organizations being listed as "terrorist." Farm Sanctuary was among them. Once we contacted the Department of Justice, our name was removed from the list. However, this has not stopped detractors from using the term, and agribusiness continues with their efforts to block us (and others) from rescuing animals in distress and exposing the conditions behind the walls and razor wire that surround factory farms. The public is starting to confront these issues, but agribusiness would rather throw up walls than invite discussions about a humane way forward. Imagine being in a business where your worst fear was that people might actually see what you're doing.

In a recently resolved case, several people entered an egg-laying facility in upstate New York owned by Wegmans, a grocery chain that operates seventy food stores in five eastern states. Wegmans sells eggs under its own label. They are produced at one of the largest egg farms in New York State, with approximately 750,000 hens. All are confined

in battery cages. Despite its reputation for supporting community initiatives where its stores are located, Wegmans denied repeated requests
from caring consumers to sell only "cage-free" eggs. It even defended
battery cages as good for the hens.

In the summer of 2004, members of the group Compassionate Consumers entered the Wegmans egg facility to document conditions inside. Their videotapes showed disturbing scenes of hens with their heads
caught in the wire mesh of their cages, submerged in manure pits, and
living in cages with dead birds. Some of the hens were unable to reach
food and water, and many had infected and untreated wounds. A few
eventually made their way to Farm Sanctuary. The activists tried to talk
to Wegmans about the shocking conditions they found, but the company refused. The activists went public.

Instead of addressing the documented problems, Wegmans tried to
defend the facility. In 2005, a company spokesperson told a Rochester,
New York, newspaper, "We feel good about our egg farm," and claimed
that it was clean and humane. Wegmans also sought prosecution of the
activists. Three charges each of criminal trespass, felony burglary, and
petty larceny were filed against Adam Durand of Compassionate Consumers. The burglary charges carried possible sentences of seven years
apiece—all for exposing brutal conditions on a factory farm.

After a three-day trial in the spring of 2006, Durand was acquitted
on the burglary charges and petty larceny and convicted only of trespass,
a misdemeanor. Despite its being Durand's first offense, the judge threw
the book at him, giving him a stiff sentence of six months in prison. In
response, Len Egert, who together with fellow attorney Amy Trakinski
represented Durand at the trial, said: "Adam's sentence was completely
excessive under the circumstances. Although the county probation department was recommending community service with no jail time, the
judge imposed the exact sentence requested by Wegmans. The influence
of agribusiness was clear." Durand's real offense, of course, was to publi-
cize the realities of factory farming. The industry responded with threats,
and the judge bowed under their pressure. Clearly the idea was to make
an example of Adam and to discourage anyone else from mounting investigations of their own.

Not only does agribusiness want to hide what's going on inside their facilities, they're doing their utmost to keep any discussion of factory farming conditions out of the public realm. Thanks to agribusiness, in many states it's a criminal offense to criticize food. These so-called food disparagement laws were invoked after Howard Lyman, a former cattle feedlot operator turned vegan, appeared on *Oprah* in 1996 to discuss the potential threat of mad cow disease in the United States. After hearing from Lyman that cows, natural herbivores, were being fed ground-up parts of cows, Oprah Winfrey said, "It has just stopped me cold from eating another burger!" A group led by Texas cattlemen sued Winfrey soon after. In 1998 a jury found in Lyman and Winfrey's favor, and the cattlemen launched a series of appeals. The final one was rejected in 2002, nearly six years after the whole episode began. The cattlemen didn't get their legal judgment, but the costly litigation case was unquestionably enough to make even powerful journalists think twice about exploring how meat is produced.

Civil Reform and Societal Change

One of the ways Farm Sanctuary is seeking to elevate the social and legal status of farm animals is through our sentient beings campaign. Chaired by Mary Tyler Moore, a longtime animal advocate who also advanced women's issues through her legendary television and film career, the campaign challenges the belief that animals are mere commodities to be exploited for food and fiber. The purpose of the effort is to get government bodies to issue proclamations that send a simple but powerful message: farm animals are sentient beings, capable of awareness, feeling, and suffering, and we humans have an ethical obligation to refrain from behaviors that inflict suffering on them.

The proclamations are largely symbolic, but their intent encapsulates our highest aims. Recognizing farm animals as sentient beings means we're obliged to provide them with more than shelter, water, and feed. The words *sentient being* also invite us to get to know farm animals and understand them in a way we never have before. As this happens, I believe people will demand an end to the abuses inherent in factory farming. I'm happy to report that the campaign has garnered support across the country. Municipalities in twenty-two states have issued official proclamations, including Little Rock, Arkansas; Tempe, Arizona; Galveston, Texas; Berkeley, California; Miami-Dade County, Florida; Dover, Delaware; Gary, Indiana; Meridian, Idaho; Houma, Louisiana; Cincinnati, Ohio; Buffalo, New York; and many others. At the federal level, senators and members of the House of Representatives are also beginning to take notice. Senator Robert Byrd of West Virginia, the longest serving senator in U.S. history, not long ago stood on the floor of the Senate and proclaimed:

> On profit-driven factory farms, veal calves are confined to dark wooden crates so small that they are prevented from lying down or scratching themselves. These creatures feel; they know pain. They suffer pain just as we humans suffer pain. Egg-laying hens are confined to battery cages. Unable to spread their wings, they are reduced to nothing more than egg-laying machines. . . . Animal cruelty abounds. It is sickening. It is infuriating. Barbaric treatment of helpless, defenseless creatures must not be tolerated even if these animals are being raised for food—and even more so, more so. Such insensitivity is insidious and can spread and is dangerous. Life must be respected and dealt with humanely in a civilized society.

U.S. representatives Peter DeFazio (D-Or.) and Christopher Shays (R-Ct.) have also taken up the challenge to provide farmed animals with some legal protection. In 2006, they introduced the Farm Animal Stewardship Purchasing Act, which would require that animal producers supplying meat, dairy products, and eggs to various federal programs—the military, prisons, school lunches, and others—comply with modest animal welfare standards. These include providing animals with sufficient shelter and space, daily access to food and water, and adequate veterinary care. Additionally, producers selling animal products to the federal government would not be permitted to starve or force-feed animals, leave sick or injured animals to languish without treatment or humane euthanasia, or confine animals so restrictively that they are unable to turn around and extend their limbs.

"Increasingly, Americans are demanding we treat farm animals more humanely," Representative DeFazio said in introducing the bill. "As a major buyer of farm animal products, the federal government can and should help lead the way, encouraging more humane practices." He's right. Although passing this bill and others like it could take years, the good news is that momentum is building. Interest in the Farm Animal Stewardship Purchasing Act is bipartisan and spans the geographic reach of the Congress. In June 2006, the Congressional Friends of Animals Caucus convened a historic hearing on farm animal welfare and discussed the DeFazio-Shays bill. It was a standing-room-only session. In his opening remarks, Representative Shays said something I heartily agree with: "The way a society treats its animals speaks to the core values and priorities of its citizens."

I spoke at the hearing, along with representatives from the Humane Society of the United States, the Animal Welfare Institute, the environmental and religious communities, and family farmers. I focused on the conditions for farmed animals in widely used confinement systems and for ducks who are force-fed to produce foie gras. I also distributed copies of *Life Behind Bars,* a Farm Sanctuary DVD narrated by Mary Tyler Moore that describes three of the most egregious confinement systems: veal crates, sow gestation crates, and hen battery cages.

I am hopeful that the U.S. public will get behind legislative reforms and reach out to their congressional representatives in large numbers, because that's what it's going to take to create changes. The agribusiness lobby is already working to make sure this doesn't happen, challenging proponents of humane reforms with menacing talk and threats of legal action. If compassionate citizens and lawmakers prevail, we will prevent untold suffering.

Progress—and Public Relations

Because farmed animals are so unprotected under U.S. law, Farm Sanctuary and other advocacy groups have to be resourceful and persistent in seeking legal remedies. Even if we don't always win, we raise awareness and educate people about factory farming's realities along the way.

In 2004, for example, we brought a landmark suit against Corcpork, California's largest pig producer. Corcpork is also known as PFFJ, which stands for "Pigs for Farmer John," Farmer John being a familiar brand in the Los Angeles area. Farmer John's slaughterhouse is located in Vernon, a few miles from downtown L.A. The exterior walls are painted with murals depicting pastoral images of happy pigs wallowing in mud and playing—a bold-faced misrepresentation of the actual conditions under which PFFJ's pigs are raised. On top of the walls barbed wire keeps intruders out.

Corcpork's facility in Corcoran houses nearly a hundred thousand pigs and is the biggest in the state. In their two-foot-wide gestation crates, Corcpork's pregnant sows have barely enough room to move, let alone turn around. They never wallow in mud or play. Our efforts to get a bill through the California legislature to ban sow crates had been torpedoed by the state's strong agribusiness lobby and legislators ready to do its bidding. But California's anti-cruelty law has a provision (penal code section 597t) requiring that anyone keeping an animal in a confined space "shall provide it [sic] with an adequate exercise area." Our lawsuit marked the first time this anti-cruelty law had been used in California to challenge a common farming practice. We weren't seeking any damages, just space for the sows to exercise a right to which they are entitled by law.

The very novelty of our suit, however, made its chances of success low, and the case was dismissed. The judge ruled that Farm Sanctuary did not have standing to bring the case on the animals' behalf.

In Arizona, we worked with a coalition of groups on a ballot initiative, the strategy successfully employed in Florida, to ban the use of both gestation and veal crates. The measure, Proposition 204, was on the November 2006 ballot, and it was approved by a 62 percent to 38 percent vote. It goes into effect in 2012. Not only will the ban improve animal welfare, it will also give Arizona's family farmers a fighting chance against massive factory farms.

As in Florida, the campaign in Arizona wasn't easy. The agribusiness lobby sought to quash the effort—and in the process grassroots, citizen-led democracy. Prior to the November 2006 vote, it tried to pass a law that would deny Arizonans the right to enact laws, such as Proposition 204, regulating agriculture and factory farming practices. That effort failed in the state legislature, but then, just months after Proposition 204 was approved by voters, agribusiness mounted other legal challenges against both the new law and Arizona's initiative process itself. I'm happy to say the Arizona law remains in place.

Also, three months after Arizonans voted to outlaw veal and gestation crates, Smithfield, the world's largest pig producer, announced plans to phase out gestation crates and replace them with group housing. Then several U.S. veal companies, including Strauss Veal, the nation's largest, announced that they would phase out veal crates. Strauss's CEO even referred to the crate system as "inhumane and archaic."

I am very happy that agribusiness is responding to public sentiments and making positive changes. However, no concrete timetable or clear plans for ending the use of gestation and veal crates have been made public, and the phase-out periods are extremely long. For instance, Smithfield estimates the pig facilities it owns outright will take ten years to complete the transition and its contract growers' facilities even longer. Despite these moves, the pigs and veal calves are still likely to be kept indoors on concrete floors, not on pasture, and will likely remain unable to express most of their natural behaviors. I am also concerned that these announcements and the related public relations efforts could be designed more to placate consumers and maintain a status quo than to reform a substantially cruel and corrupt system. Going forward, we will have to monitor the situation closely.

We're working on a citizen initiative in California that aims to ban veal crates, gestation crates, and for the first time ever, battery cages. Dedicated volunteers took to the streets and collected nearly 500,000 signatures of citizens to qualify the measure for the November 2008 ballot. If successful, it will mandate that calves raised for veal, sows used for breeding, and hens exploited in egg production be given at least enough space to turn around and stretch their limbs.

In 2007, we celebrated another encouraging development when Wolfgang Puck, the Los Angeles–based celebrity chef whose empire includes restaurants, catering operations, and a range of frozen foods, said that he would no longer sell foie gras. He will also be offering more vegan options. "We decided about three months ago to be really much more socially responsible," Puck told *The New York Times*. "We feel the quality of the food is better, and our conscience feels better." Farm Sanctuary and our supporters had been reaching out to Puck for years on these issues, and we were very pleased with these developments.

Not all of the legal action for farmed animal welfare is taking place out west. In 1996, the New Jersey state legislature amended New Jersey's anti-cruelty statute to require the state Department of Agriculture to draft and adopt humane standards for the treatment of domestic livestock. They were supposed to do this within six months, but the deadline came and went. Seven long years later the standards were finally released, but they included a sweeping exemption for industry practices "commonly taught" by veterinary schools and other agricultural institutions. The regulations allowed the use of gestation crates for sows and forced molting (starvation) of laying hens. Agribusiness had a large hand in the drafting process. When it came to language pertaining to veal calves, for instance, the department incorporated the words of the American Veal Association directly into the standards and claimed these were humane.

The new standards were weak, to say the least, and even restricted the role of the enforcement authority of the state SPCA. They no longer reflected the mandate of the state legislature, and so, in 2005, Farm Sanctuary joined with a broad coalition of humane organizations, farmers, veterinarians, and environmental and consumer groups to ask the courts to overturn New Jersey farming regulations. This effort is of particular concern given our unsuccessful attempt to convict a New Jersey egg factory for discarding live hens in a trash can. The company's attorney actually argued in court that the birds could legally be treated like manure.

The New Jersey challenge goes beyond any previous legal action taken on behalf of farm animals in that it seeks a judicial declaration that most common factory farming practices are inhumane and, therefore, illegal under New Jersey law. The case is ongoing and has been taken up by the state's supreme court. New Jersey remains the only state in the country that explicitly requires a code of humane standards for farm animals. So there's a unique opportunity there to improve farm animals' quality of life while influencing similar humane measures nationwide. It's important that New Jersey residents make their voices heard and let the department know that humane standards should not codify cruelty to animals as legal and acceptable farming practice.

A Horrible Hors d'Oeuvre

One of our most intense recent legal efforts has been to ban the forced feeding of geese and ducks to produce the expensive French-derived *pâté de foie gras* (in French, *foie gras* means "fatty liver"). French can lend an air of sophistication to food, but the truth is that bringing this luxury item to dining tables entails enormous quantities of grain and a great big dose of cruelty.

The United States has three foie gras facilities, two in New York and one in California, which together produce about eight hundred thousand pounds of duck liver a year. In France, geese are also force-fed, although ducks are more commonly the victims simply because they are cheaper to raise. In the United States, the industry has centered on ducks, about twenty-four million of whom are killed each year for meat, foie gras, and feathers. Most are raised in factory farms, where they are denied fresh air, freedom of movement, and water for bathing.

Foie gras production is particularly unsavory. At just a few months old, ducks are confined inside dark sheds with hundreds of others. Here they are force-fed enormous amounts of food several times a day. A farm worker grabs the ducks and, one by one, thrusts a pipe down their throats so that a corn mixture can be driven directly into their gullets. Generally this lasts between two weeks and a month, during which time the ducks become grossly overweight. Their livers expand up to ten times their normal size—growing diseased and dysfunctional—and then the ducks are slaughtered.

Not surprisingly given their girth and treatment, ducks raised for foie gras have difficulty standing, walking, and even breathing, as their engorged livers crowd their other internal organs. Many suffer traumatic injuries as they are handled and the rigid pipe is shoved quickly down their esophagus. Necropsies performed on foie gras ducks have shown extreme obesity, impaction of undigested food in the esophagus, lacerations in the throat, and a proliferation of bacterial and fungal growth in their upper digestive tracts. Many die before the feeding cycle ends. Indeed, the mortality rate for ducks raised on foie gras farms is among the highest in the farming industry.

No matter how industry apologists try to spin it, there is simply no humane way to produce foie gras. Even in Europe, where foie gras still has many defenders, opposition is growing, including in France. Several European countries, including Italy and Poland, have outlawed force-feeding of ducks or geese, and the EU is considering a unionwide ban. Israel's supreme court recently found that forced feeding was "violent and harmful" and violated the anti-cruelty law, thereby effectively outlawing the production of foie gras. Even Pope Benedict XVI has weighed in on the issue. The then Cardinal Joseph Ratzinger replied to a German journalist's question on animal welfare this way: animals, he said, are our "companions in creation," to whom we owe moral consideration. "Certainly, a sort of industrial use of creatures, so that geese are fed in such a way as to produce as large a liver as possible, or hens live so packed together that they become just caricatures of birds, this degrading of living creatures to a commodity seems to me in fact to contradict the relationship of mutuality that comes across in the Bible."

Awareness of the horrors of force-feeding birds to make foie gras is increasing. When they learn about it, most Americans oppose the cruelty of foie gras. This has encouraged a number of efforts to ban its production and sale in the United States. In 2004, California made the force-feeding of ducks and geese for foie gras and its sale illegal, the first state in the United States to do so. California's historic law goes into effect in 2012.

On the heels of California's action came another victory. In April 2006, Chicago's City Council voted to ban the sale of foie gras. This was another major advance for farmed animals. That it happened in the city poet Carl Sandburg called the "hog butcher for the world" is particularly sweet.

Like a growing number of efforts to improve farm animal welfare, the campaign to ban the sale of foie gras in Chicago brought together a diverse group of legislators, businesses, organizations, religious groups, and individuals. One of these individuals was Jana Kohl, a psychologist and longtime animal advocate who is also a member of the well-known family that founded the Kohl's department stores. She's also the niece of U.S. senator Herb Kohl of Wisconsin. Jana was a tireless advocate and educator. She put together packets of information on foie gras and met with many aldermen to explain the need for the ban. While we all came from different perspectives, we found common ground on the principle that diners' enjoyment of foie gras couldn't justify the price the ducks pay to provide it.

A war of words between two of the city's best-known chefs also fueled publicity for our effort. The whole thing began a few years back when Farm Sanctuary worked on a bill in the Illinois legislature to ban foie gras production. Agribusiness interests stopped the bill's progress, but the issue got some media attention. In turn, this led to a blow-up, played out in Chicago's famously feisty press, between celebrity chef Charlie Trotter, who in the interest of treating animals humanely doesn't serve foie gras in his namesake Chicago restaurant, and chef Rick Tramonto, who does. The chefs' back-and-forth caught the attention of Alderman Joe Moore and educated him about what's involved in producing foie gras. Soon after, he introduced a measure before the City Council to ban its sale.

Alderman Moore's proposal was assigned to the council's health committee, which gave it a good chance of being passed. Of course, the foie gras industry did their best to derail the bill, although those testifying on their behalf weren't very convincing. The foie gras producers sent out their top experts to the hearings, including a former USDA veterinarian. At one point, the committee chair cut off a stem-winder by the vet. "Now give me a straight answer," he said. "Is your specialty animal husbandry?"

The "expert" had to answer truthfully. "No sir," was the reply.

The manager of Hudson Valley Foie Gras, a producer in New York State, also testified, unconvincingly, that force-feeding was no big deal for the ducks. A Chicago chef and restaurant owner, Didier Durand, offered his opinion that the consumption of foie gras in the region of southern France where he was born was the reason cholesterol levels and heart attack rates there are the lowest in France. Most of the council members looked at him in utter disbelief, as did I.

The ban also had many supporters. I testified in its favor, as did actress Loretta Swit, a long-time animal advocate. Loretta's of Polish extraction, and Chicago has a large Polish American community. She also has ties to the city from her work over the years, and she spoke passionately in favor of the ban. We provided scientific evidence of the ducks' suffering, photos of what the animals go through, and a number of testimonials. These came from, among others, veterinarian Holly Cheever, who has visited foie gras facilities, once with a representative of Whole Foods Market. Whole Foods had considered selling foie gras but was so appalled by what it discovered that it abandoned those plans.

After months of deliberation, the health committee passed the bill overwhelmingly and sent it to the full City Council for its consideration. The night after the committee's vote, Durand's restaurant was vandalized and animal rights "extremists" were blamed. We were extremely skeptical: the timing seemed too perfect. I don't believe the vandalism was perpetrated by anybody within the animal-protection community. Committing violence is the antithesis of all that Farm Sanctuary and the animal rights movement stands for. Happily, the incident didn't get much attention in the press, and we were able to keep the discussion focused on the facts of foie gras production.

On April 26, 2006, the City Council was scheduled to vote on the ban, and all of us involved in the effort felt enormous anxiety. We were going up or we were going down, and the vote could swing either way. Any one of Chicago's aldermen might speak out loudly against the proposal and sink the ban. (Even lawmakers can get emotional about these issues.) The tension was palpable when Alderman Ed Smith, chair of the health committee and a supporter of Moore's humane measure, brought the legislation up and announced that he wanted to add it to the omnibus bill. "Is there any discussion?" the chairman of the council asked. We waited. Silence. There was no further discussion. The facts had spoken for themselves. The ban was added to the omnibus bill, which passed by a vote of forty-eight to one. It was astounding. I believe what happened that morning in Chicago was confirmation that we all share a deeply held revulsion against cruelty to other animals, even if we don't always give voice to our feelings.

Soon after the vote, a group of us who had worked on the ban went to a restaurant across the street from City Hall and celebrated with champagne (Jana Kohl's gift). It was a sunny spring day, so after lunch, Jana and I and her dog, Baby, went for a walk in Lincoln Park, processing the whole experience along the way. Eventually, we sat on a bench near a big pond full of geese and ducks swimming, diving, and flying—the perfect end to a very good day.

* * *

Almost as soon as the Chicago bill passed, the U.S. foie gras industry began their rollback campaign. It created a trade association and hired lobbyists and political operatives to challenge the Chicago law and represent its interests with legislators across the United States. Some restaurateurs in Chicago have been flouting the ban, calling the law silly and denigrating those who worked to enact it. We've responded by stating that cruelty to animals is a serious matter that often indicates broader societal problems, and it should not be ignored or dismissed.

Sadly, in 2008 Chicago's foie gras ban was repeated when Mayor Daley and his cronies on the city council pulled a fast one. They rushed the repeal ordinance through committee and the council floor on the same day, without a hearing. And they refused to allow anybody to speak in opposition. I consider their actions an affront to both animal welfare and the democratic process. I also understand foie gras producers are creating a strategic plan to gain more government-sanctioned, institutional support. They have already scored one victory. In summer 2006, New York governor George Pataki authorized more than $400,000 of taxpayers' money to help Hudson Valley Foie Gras expand its production. We're trying to stop such subsidies and will continue pressing the matter.

The foie gras issue ultimately comes down to the question of where you draw the line. As I told USA Today a few weeks after the Chicago vote in 2006, foie gras is merely an appetizer. "It's gustatory narcissism," I said. "What are we willing to do for this flavor?" For those who want to eat pâté, there are many alternatives, including "faux gras" made with mushrooms, walnuts, and rosemary, and spinach and pimento pâté. The force-feeding of ducks and geese crosses a line, as do other egregious factory farming cruelties, such as veal and gestation crates and battery cages. Critics of animal welfare reforms always ask, "Where will it end? What's next?" Those are exactly the questions I ask about unnecessarily cruel treatment of farm animals. Where does *that* end? What are the limits of animal exploitation? And at what point do we demand basic standards of conduct?

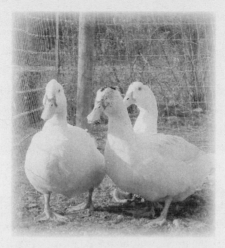

Burton, Harper, and Kohl

PROFILE: Burton, Kohl, and Harper

In late October 2005, four ducks from a foie gras facility were left on the porch of the Watkins Glen shelter. They were in bad shape. One was missing an eye, two others had crippled legs, and all four were breathing through open mouths—a bad sign for a duck and in all likelihood the result of their huge livers pressing up against their lungs. With the ducks were photos and videos taken inside the facility. The images showed dead ducks in cages and live, injured ones. One of the four rescued ducks had a bloody chest and legs, possibly from the trauma of handling or from scraping against the cage's floor and walls. Ducks' livers can get so large that the animals can no longer move and may suffer broken legs. It was obvious none of the four had gotten veterinary care.

One of our staff members agreed to drive the ducks, who were named Burton, Kohl, Harper, and Damon, to Cornell. The Cornell vets diagnosed the ducks with hepatic lipidosis, or fatty liver syndrome. Shocking, isn't it? When people eat foie gras, they're really eating a diseased product. The vets prescribed antibiotics and also recommended natural remedies, such as the herb milk thistle, that would help heal the ducks' livers. Sadly, Damon's legs were so severely crippled that the vets recommended he be euthanized. As with all such decisions, it was a difficult one.

Initially, the three surviving ducks were scared of people and showed it by being less than friendly. For two months, as their wounds healed, they had to be hand-fed. It was as if they'd lost their knowledge of how to eat or their interest in it as a result of being force-fed. But this method of feeding was far gentler than the foie gras industry's. Instead of stiff metal, the feeding tube was flexible plastic, very thin, and lubricated. The tube was inserted slowly into the ducks' mouths, accompanied by calming words and feather stroking. Industry defenders like to say that the ducks waddle up for food or eagerly come to the front of their cages. Not these ducks! They clearly hated it and generally tried to avoid people at mealtimes. It was as if they thought, "Oh, great, another force-feeder!"

When Burton, Kohl, and Harper finally began to eat on their own, the staffer taking care of them said she felt like playing a recording of the "Hallelujah Chorus" from Handel's *Messiah*. Happily, the trio is now healthy. All three are gentle, and each is a character. Burton, who's the biggest, is macho and the most independent. He likes hanging out with other ducks. Harper, the one who's missing an eye, is sweet-natured. He had a beak malformation, so his head is a little lopsided, but he doesn't seem to have any neurological problems. He likes to cuddle and wrap his neck around you. Kohl, because of his malformed leg, walks on his elbows and is clearly the baby of the group.

CHAPTER THIRTEEN

Beneath the Skin

I recently saw the traveling exhibition "Bodies," a series of galleries full of preserved human cadavers with their skin removed to show muscles, tissues, organs, and bones displayed in various poses that reveal how our anatomy functions. I was struck by how intensely interested the other visitors were in the internal workings of the human form. I too was fascinated by the startlingly beautiful complexity of our bodies. We could also see lungs blackened by smoke and arteries clogged with plaque. The diseased cadavers were no random happenstance, as the exhibit's booklet explained: "It is widely reported in the national press that too many people are overweight, that many preventable medical conditions, such as heart disease and certain forms of cancer, are on the increase and that exorbitant costs of medical insurance and hospital care continue to rise." It concluded: "Today it seems that the best medicine anyone could possibly prescribe to get at the root cause of these problems is a good dose of body education."

When I think about it, giving "a good dose of body education" is what I've been trying to do over the last twenty years. It was self-evident to those of us at the exhibition that day that our muscles and flesh aren't all that different from those of cows, pigs, lambs, and the other animals we eat. One of the bodies on display was sliced into cross sections. The thighs were cut in round segments about as thick as steaks with a reddish-colored flesh surrounding the bone. In other specimens, "meat" was separated from the bone and looked unmistakably like beef filets. The exhibition confirmed for me how very vulnerable as well as mysterious and indeed miraculous all animals are. It also reminded me how disconnected we humans can be from ourselves and others. Sad to say, we're capable of causing great harm to ourselves and others through ignorance and carelessness.

I couldn't help overhearing people making connections between what they put in their bodies and what their bodies looked like, between their bodies and those of other animals. More and more, I see people making this connection and then deciding to change their lives. I want to explore some of these connections—in the corporate world, in the body politic, and within individuals—and offer suggestions for how you can give yourself a "good dose of body education." (As an appendix, I've included a Resources section with books, websites, and organizations that will provide further useful information.)

Resistance and Reconnection

If you've read this book from start to finish, you've gotten more than just a glimpse of the colossal cruelty of industrial farming. You've also read about how dominant agribusiness is as a force in the United States today. Its practices cut corners and violate values of sustainability that farmers abided by in the past. Those values—such as integrity and honesty—are perhaps why some farmers are questioning the direction of agriculture. An emerging interest in more sustainable, smaller-scale farming, coupled with powerful community and individual actions, is starting to reshape the landscape of U.S. food production. I don't have the space here to describe all the micro-enterprises and movements that are underway, so a few examples will have to suffice.

In Iowa, the largest pig-producing state in the country, the Animal Welfare Institute is working with family farmers who have rejected the factory-farm model and who are returning to a more traditional family farm model. I've also heard about Iowa soybean growers who've gotten out of the business of selling feed for pigs altogether. Instead they grow organic soybeans, which they sell to tofu producers at premium prices. In 2003, the American Public Health Association joined the debate about industrial farming. It called for a moratorium on new factory farms and further research into the health impacts of air and water pollution produced by existing facilities.

Residents of Williams County, Ohio, have formed an alliance to prevent the construction of a five-million-chicken mega-farm in the county. A representative of the Ohio Farmers' Union told the people fighting the factory farm, "What you are confronting is a very distinct change in the history of your county," and noted that the spread of CAFOs was putting the culture of family farming and the environment at risk. In 2001, the city of Tulsa, Oklahoma, sued the poultry industry after algae blooms tied to the manure from Arkansas chicken facilities polluted Tulsa's water supply. You read that right—the volume of chicken waste is so enormous that significant portions of it made its way from northwest Arkansas into Oklahoma. In 2005, the state of Oklahoma sued poultry operations for pollution from their facilities that had fouled the Illinois River water basin, a popular recreation area.

Pockets of resistance are cropping up across the United States. Citizens near our farm at Watkins Glen recently joined forces to combat a Pennsylvania feed company that was inviting struggling farmers to sign contracts to raise pigs in factory farm conditions. Hundreds of citizens, including me, attended public meetings where we stood together against corporate farming.

At one event, a representative from the Farm Bureau extolled the benefits of contract growing but wasn't able to address prospective farmers' concerns about losing control of their own means of production and becoming dependent on an out-of-state corporation. As I looked around the hall, I recognized several familiar faces, including a dairy farmer who'd been critical of Farm Sanctuary in the past. I assumed he'd be supportive of the bureau's agenda, but after I raised my hand and asked a question about whether large hog factories could present a pollution problem, he handed me a note describing his own worries about polluted water. Over the course of that meeting, we passed that piece of paper back and forth, sharing our observations and common concerns. In spite of our history on opposite sides of the debate about the farming of animals, we both believed that our part of New York State, with its beautiful lakes, rivers, gorges, and waterfalls, should be protected.

The battle in rural New York continues. Although a number of towns in the Finger Lakes region have sought to regulate the construction of factory farms, the New York State Department of Agriculture and Markets, which like other state agriculture departments is a defender of factory farming, has threatened the towns with lawsuits under the state's right-to-farm law. Some towns have withdrawn their opposition in the face of this pressure, and we don't yet know what the outcome will be. What is certain is that public officials give up fighting for the interests of family farmers and the community too often. Ironically, it's the animal rights or environmental activists, or busybody do-gooders, who are often blamed for supposedly restricting farmers from doing business as it "should be" done.

Another form of resistance to industrialized farming is the growth of organic farming. In the past decade it's been one of the fastest-growing sectors of U.S. agriculture. The area devoted to organic cropland doubled between 1992 and 1997 and, for many crops, doubled again between 1997 and 2003. Sales of organic poultry and dairy have increased by about 20 percent each year since 1997, a rate that continues as of this writing. (In comparison, during the same period, sales of all food in the United States rose only 2 to 4 percent a year.) In 2005, sales of organic foods in the United States were nearly $14 billion. That's about 2.5 percent of the total retail market for food, still just a fraction of the astounding $894 billion Americans spent on food in 2005.

This explosion of demand has not been lost on corporate America. Large companies have been buying up smaller organic food manufacturers and moving into the market for vegan and vegetarian products. Kraft now owns Boca Burger, makers of a popular veggie burger; Kellogg's bought Kashi, a whole-grain-cereal company; Dean Foods, a major dairy company, owns Silk soy milk; and ConAgra, a giant agribusiness company, owns Lightlife, which produces a range of vegan meat substitutes, including Tofu Pups, Smart Dogs, Smart Deli Slices, and Fakin' bacon. As a result, a wider variety of foods free of animal products and toxic chemicals is now available throughout the country and, increasingly, in mainstream supermarkets.

While the interest of corporations has made vegan "meats" and organic foods more easily accessible, it has also led to wider availability of organic animal products. Unfortunately the organic label does not necessarily mean improvements in animal welfare. On farms that are certified as organic, the animals are fed grain or grass that does not contain pesticides. They are not routinely injected with hormones or antibiotics. But they can still be intensively farmed and confined.

This is why consumers concerned with animal welfare should be skeptical about the organic label. It does not guarantee that the animals were treated well, were allowed to express their natural behaviors, and had as painless a death as possible. Likewise, too many of the "humane" claims on meat and dairy products reflect the producers' interest in marketing its product rather than earnest adherence to principles of animal welfare. A good number of them are a sham. A recent article on the front page of *The New York Times'* Dining and Wine section, "Be It Ever So Homespun, There's Nothing Like Spin," points to a growing number of product labels claiming that foods are produced in a responsible manner. But, as the article documents, many of these labels are examples of what's called "greenwashing" and do not accurately reflect the reality behind them. As a consumer, you'll have to dig deeper for more information. I suggest you cast a skeptical eye on such claims until you learn more about whether they're accurate or not. Product labels with pictures of happy animals are no guarantee that the animals were treated well.

Indeed, the Wisconsin-based Cornucopia Institute, which represents small farming interests, recently brought a lawsuit to require that cows whose milk was being sold as organic be given space to graze. The suit was directed at Horizon and Aurora, the two largest organic milk producers. In response, Whole Foods Market's founder, John Mackey, was quoted in *The New York Times* as saying, "We think the average customer believes organic dairy cows are grazing full time . . . and we would like organic standards to be more rigorous so the perception meets the reality."

Some corporations are starting to take the issue of animal welfare seriously. After pressure from advocates, McDonald's has instituted a number of measures to ensure a minimum of animal welfare in its products, while Burger King (nationwide) and McDonald's (in selected cities) have put veggie burgers on their menu. A major player in the organic foods industry, Whole Foods Market, the world's largest retailer of natural and organic foods, has taken some important steps to promote animal welfare in recent years. Founded in 1980 in Austin, Texas, Whole Foods went public in 1992 and has grown to become a $5.7 billion company, with hundreds of stores across the United States and in Britain. It recently announced plans to acquire Wild Oats, the second-largest U.S. natural foods retailer. After witnessing inhumane conditions at a foic gras farm, Whole Foods officials pledged in 1997 not to sell this cruel product. In 2006, Whole Foods decided not to carry live lobsters in its stores, and under John Mackey's leadership it is developing standards that seek to better address farmed animals' physical, emotional, and behavioral needs. Mackey became especially concerned about the cruelty of industrialized production after hearing about it at a shareholders' meeting from an animal rights campaigner, Lauren Ornelas, who was urging the company not to sell factory-farmed duck meat. The idea is to set an example of responsible corporate citizenship, and create a better standard for how to raise animals. It is Mackey's vision that in twenty years these standards will help raise awareness and make factory farming a thing of the past.

I am under no illusion that Whole Foods Market is likely to become a vegan company, even though John Mackey himself is basically a vegan (with the exception of the eggs he eats from his own free-roaming hens). However, if Whole Foods' efforts can help make more transparent the egregious animal abuse that has become rampant on factory farms, then this is a positive step forward (during speeches, Mackey sometimes shows a video to make this point). Whole Foods Market has also made a commitment to sell more locally produced foods and is setting up a program to offer loans to small organic farmers. I hope that partnerships such as these will grow and will, with other efforts, help turn the tide against cruel industrial farming.

Returning to Agrarian Roots

Although the rapid growth of organic farming is a welcome sign, many people active in the local and organic foods movements have expressed concerns about large corporations dominating the market and squeezing out small producers. Since these are concerns I share, I'm encouraged by the resurgence of small farms and farmers' markets I see when I travel around the country.

One of the most exciting local and community-organized projects is

CSAs, or community-supported agriculture programs, which came to the United States in the early 1990s. What began with a handful of producers has now grown to encompass more than a thousand operations, and the numbers continue to rise. CSAs provide a mechanism for people to invest directly in food production by paying a sum of money up front to a farm and receiving produce over the course of the season. The customers share the risks with the farmer and receive fresh, seasonal, and organic produce in return. It is a positive model that connects farmers with consumers and helps engender an understanding between the two. CSAs also promise a future for rural communities, where the past few decades have seen farm after farm give way to real estate development or foreclosure and farmers' children leave for the city.

Like CSAs, farmers' markets allow consumers to communicate directly with farmers and understand our dependency on the earth and those who grow what we eat. Farmers' markets exist in every state. There's even one in the town of North Pole, Alaska. I recently visited the Hollywood Farmers' Market with my mother. As we walked around together, we admired the many booths that offered simply packaged and prepared foods: dried fruits and nuts, baked goods, cooked greens, tasty vegan stews, burritos, and falafel. Coffee, tea, and various juices were also available. Food vendors gave out free samples, and shoppers happily partook of them and told the producers what they thought.

Since it began in 1993, the Hollywood market has grown to accommodate hundreds of vendors and thousands of visitors every week, and it continues to expand. The name may make it sound like a gathering place for the rich and famous, but like other farmers' markets, it is frequented by many working-class folks of average means. Farmers come from throughout California to sell their wares there. One who sells a variety of organic fruits told me that there was a long waiting list for booths, but the truth is it's more than a collection of booths—it's a real community meeting place. The outdoor market is full of musicians of all ages playing instruments, singing, selling CDs, and even dancing. Artisans sell paintings, frames, and textiles, along with plants both edible and decorative. Everywhere you look there's commercial activity, and all of the products are vitally connected to the community that created them.

I know that many Americans still live from paycheck to paycheck in neighborhoods that are virtually food deserts, and that's a shame. Healthy and sustainable foods should be available for everyone, not just people of means. The Hollywood farmers' market has gotten this message. With its partners—the USDA, the University of California at Los Angeles, and Los Angeles County—the market offers a master gardener volunteer training program to help low-income communities grow and eat more nutritious food. The partnership hopes to create a host of micro-entrepreneurs who will bring the message of health and sustainability to every part of the Los Angeles area.

Across the country in New York City, demand for fresh, local produce is strong and growing. There are now more than forty-five greenmarkets in the city's five boroughs, supplied by nearly two hundred farmers from New York and surrounding states. The growers staff their booths, which feature a variety of crops, including asparagus and rhubarb in the spring, peaches and corn in the summer, and pumpkins and pears in the fall. With more than seventy vendors, one of New York City's most active greenmarket locations is in Manhattan's Union Square. On a cold winter weekend a few years back, I paid them a visit. Despite the freezing weather and blizzard predictions, farmers and bakers were doing a decent business. I bought a cup of hot apple cider and a cup of freshly squeezed wheatgrass juice from a Brooklyn grower.

Greenmarkets also give City Harvest—an organization that supports community food programs—hundreds of thousands of pounds of food each year to feed New York's hungry. The director of greenmarkets told me that demand for fresh, local produce was strong and growing. In fact, he said, they needed more farmers to provide it. This integration of city with country offers a dynamic paradigm that can improve people's health in urban areas and revitalize struggling rural communities with many small farms and diverse crops. Some greenmarket farmers accept food stamps, which helps people of all means to have access to healthy, locally produced food.

Strolling around the farmers' markets on both coasts, I was struck by the contrast between shopping there and shopping at a supermarket. Goods at these greenmarkets are not chemical-laden, repackaged, over-processed, or shipped great distances to be put on a shelf or in a case in an anonymous store under artificial light. Instead, here was public space given over to the expression of community—a marketplace of food and arts and crafts and ideas, where people stopped and spoke with each other and where grower and consumer could meet. By contrast, super-markets feel almost like a race to stockpile resources and elbow your way to the shortest checkout line, where a cashier swipes your purchases over a scanner as you peruse the tabloids and candy selection. As we push the shopping cart around the overly air-conditioned aisles, how often do we stop to remember the soil the food came from, the sun that shone and the rain that fell, or the animals whose lives were taken to feed us? How often do we stop and talk with our fellow shoppers about the food?

Nowhere, perhaps, is our connection to the land and our bodies more immediate than in community gardens. These urban oases offer city people the chance to grow food and build community at the same time. Of course, a community garden doesn't have to be in the city. We have a garden at the shelter at Watkins Glen, and I've spent hours there discussing large and small issues with friends while pulling weeds, plant-ing seeds, sampling fresh greens, or tilling the soil by hand. It's honest and straightforward work, and creates a sense of belonging.

These gardens can also show us the meaning of generosity. At harvest time, our gardens typically produce more than we can consume, so we give part of our harvest away and graciously accept our neighbors' over-flow. Throughout the summer, tomatoes, cucumbers, squash, beans, and other produce harvested from backyard gardens are left on the kitchen table at Farm Sanctuary's main office, free for the taking. The goodness of the earth becomes shared bounty. Community gardens also teach us the value of growing food where we live and appreciating our regions' natural and cultural diversity. This is what the Slow Food movement is all about: taking the time to enjoy the pleasures of food with friends or family, protecting food from the homogenization of fast-food culture, and supporting agricultural biodiversity. Founded in Italy in 1986, Slow Food has now spread to over a hundred countries. It's something I sup-port, except when it involves the exploitation of animals.

I believe we can create a truly humane, sustainable, and healthy food production system without killing any animals. I imagine a revolution in veganic agriculture in which small farmers grow a variety of vegetables, fruits, grains, and legumes, all fertilized with vegetable sources. Farms such as these have the potential to revitalize once-thriving farming communities across America. One of the reasons people over the ages have raised animals, especially in cold climates, is that crops don't grow in the winter. But I think there is money to be made in value-added products such as preserves (jams, chutneys, etc.) and roots stored in cellars, while other parts of the country that are warmer year-round can provide the foods that northern climates cannot sustain. I can also envision a future where every home comes equipped with a small greenhouse so that fruits and vegetables can be grown throughout the winter. Even in apartments, people can grow tomatoes, peppers, and herbs on their windowsills, on fire escapes, or even on "green" roofs.

Farm Sanctuary is constantly looking for allies concerned about the planet and those who live upon it. Increasingly, we are working with environmental, health, community, sustainable farming, religious, consumer, and various other organizations, all of which recognize the ties we have to the land and the importance of sustainable agriculture and family farms.

A Kinder Plate

The best and easiest way to promote health, compassion, and sustainability is to adopt a vegan lifestyle and to buy locally produced, organic plant foods. Animal foods, including meat, milk, and eggs, waste vast resources and are inherently violent. I know that no agricultural system is completely harmless, including strictly vegetarian ones. The very act of living on this earth means we impact and unintentionally hurt others. Indeed, a born-again Christian friend of mine believes that "something must die so that we can live." I don't necessarily disagree with this, if we consider plants living beings. But I wholly reject the notion that animals must die for us to live. Eating plants instead of animals goes a long way toward promoting kindness and sustainability, not to mention good health.

Becoming a vegan is not about self-denial; it's more a matter of self-awareness. It is about trying new foods and broadening your palate, expressing the joy of being alive, and knowing that you're making a daily effort to live less violently and more sustainably. Being vegan is defined by a sense of care and responsibility to the land and life around us. It's a principled refusal to add to the violence of the world, and an intention to be a witness for something better. All we're really talking about is living with compassion and integrity and aspiring to be the best we can be, just as we all try to do in other areas of life.

If becoming vegan overnight seems too difficult, then try it every other day, or once a week. Eating vegan meals doesn't have to be complicated. In fact, it's becoming easier than ever, and meals can be as plain or as fancy as you wish. There are a host of guides on going vegan and many vegan cookbooks, along with numerous websites that can help you make nutritious as well as humane decisions about what to put on your plate. There are all kinds of non-meat and non-dairy alternatives to your favorite foods, and I have included some sources of these in the Resources section. It goes without saying that it is possible to be a vegan and not eat a balanced diet, just as it is possible to be an omnivore and not get adequate nutrition. It's important to eat a diet rich in whole foods, including fruits, vegetables, nuts, grains, and legumes, to cut out destructive health practices (such as smoking or drinking to excess), and enhance positive lifestyles (such as regular exercise and practicing yoga or meditation).

But don't take just my word for it. A respected group of health professionals at the American Dietetic Association has this to say: "Well-planned vegan and other types of vegetarian diets are appropriate for all stages of the life cycle, including during pregnancy, lactation, infancy, childhood and adolescence. Vegetarian diets offer a number of nutritional benefits, including lower levels of saturated fat, cholesterol, and animal protein as well as higher levels of carbohydrates, fiber, magnesium, potassium, folate, and antioxidants such as vitamins C and E and phytochemicals."

If you continue eating meat and dairy products and you are concerned about animal welfare, then I hope you'll avoid factory-farmed meat, milk, and eggs. To buy these products is to shore up a system of abuse that destroys animals and people, ecosystems, and healthy communities. Every time we spend a dollar on food we are effectively saying, "I support this system."

Another word of advice: think critically. Challenge assumptions and so-called conventional wisdom. Ask questions, and go to a trusted source for information. Talk to farmers and develop an understanding of how they produce what they're selling. At supermarkets, food co-ops, and health food stores, you can ask about how and where the food in your basket was grown or raised. As you do this, you'll become more informed, and you'll also let producers know they'll be held to account for their practices. If you get a superficial answer or if there's resistance to sharing this kind of information, consider shopping somewhere else.

The only way to know with certainty how farm animals are treated is to visit the farm where your meat, dairy, or eggs came from. A number of farmers who sell their products at farmers' markets open their doors certain days of the year. If the owner has nothing to hide, then he or she should welcome your interest. If he or she doesn't allow consumers to see the farm's operations, be skeptical about the conditions for the animals. Even if you *are* welcomed, dig deeper. Find out what happens to the male calves born on dairies. Do they spend time with their mothers? Ask how old the animals are when they are sent to slaughter. How confident is the farmer that the slaughterhouse renders the animals unconscious before slaughter? The closer you can get to the source of your food, the better, because there's greater accountability. The further you're removed from food, the easier it is for producers to hide poor practices and irresponsible behaviors. It is this disconnect that has allowed factory farming to spread.

Above all, I encourage you to become involved in decisions about your food. Show up at community meetings; join your local CSA or food cooperative or start one. Shop at your farmers' market, buy local and/or organic produce, visit a pick-your-own farm, or even grow your own. Share the bounty. Learn from the cows: chew your food carefully, ruminate, and experience what you're eating. Not only is this pleasurable, it actually helps your body digest the nutrients in food more thoroughly. Eating is supposed to satisfy our hunger and nourish our bodies, and when we eat well it does. Food can also delight our senses. Cool fruit is a refreshing antidote to the summer heat, just as a warm bowl of soup can take the chill off a cold winter day.

Expand your palate to enjoy the richness of the plant world—the seasons' gifts. Encouraging this in the young is the mission of Antonia Demas, a Cornell Ph.D. who has pioneered a school curriculum that combines food, nutrition, culture, and the arts. Through it, children can explore and enjoy the textures and colors of plant foods: the yellows, reds, greens, purples, oranges, and everything in between. Demas founded the Food Studies Institute and has been working to encourage schools to include more healthy, plant-based options in their menus so our kids get nutritious lunches, not brand-name junk stuffed with empty calories.

When you eat out, go to places that promote local food and a respect for the earth. More and more restaurants are beginning to specialize in locally produced foods. Many are growing their own herbs and vegetables, sometimes shortening the journey from field to table to a matter of feet! I encourage you to visit these places often. If your favorite restaurant doesn't serve local produce or healthy meals, ask the manager why not, and whether it's possible to do so. If you eat at fast-food restaurants, and many of us do (over the last thirty years our spending on fast food has increased a staggering eighteen times, from $6 billion to $110 billion a year), make a point of choosing the salads and the veggie burgers. You'll give your dollars a voice in support of healthier and more sustainable meals, and you'll give the franchise a reason to expand similar offerings.

If you're worried about the cost of food, consider this: the more processed or full of chemicals the product (think chicken nuggets, hot dogs, and hamburgers), the more likely it is that the costs of that product have been externalized or hidden. It's also more likely that unsustainable or cruel behavior went into producing it. In other words, if the food is cheap and highly processed, there's probably a reason why.

U.S. farmers are proud of saying that in this country less than 10 percent of what we spend goes toward food, the lowest proportion of anywhere in the world. By contrast, in 1930, nearly one-third of Americans' income was used to purchase food. Today, even as we're saving money at the checkout counter, we're losing it in environmental and community degradation, the taste and nutrition of our food, and the growing costs of health care. Why is our food so full of chemical additives and preservatives? Why are convenience foods so full of fat and sugar? Why do we stuff ourselves with cheap food that ultimately satisfies so little of our nutritional needs? Why does producing our food lead to massive air and water pollution and huge quantities of toxic waste? Why are popular foods leading us ever further into national crises of obesity and diabetes?

We have to ask ourselves whether the multiple costs of cheap food are worth it, and answer honestly.

There are many ways to squeeze more value out of our food dollars. Increasing numbers of communities across the United States are setting up urban gardens for growing vegetables and fruit, making healthy produce affordable and available. Many of these have strong links to schools or youth programs. Food dollars could be better spent on a sack of potatoes instead of potato chips.

Of course, we have to work to make healthy foods more widely available in poor communities. When I was in Washington, D.C., I lived in a pretty tough part of town, and it was hard to get good food. The corner grocery store had cookies, soda, and lots of other junk food, but almost nothing fresh or healthy. I'd like to see these stores stock more fruits and vegetables, including those grown locally. Buying clubs where people get together and purchase in bulk are another option.

The United States can boast of a beautiful mosaic of cultures and food traditions, yet somehow we've bought into the idea of the hamburger as our national food. So many traditional cuisines are largely plant-based and provide us with all the nutrients we need. Why not reclaim these food roots and share our cultural heritage? Our bodies and our communities would be the healthier for it.

The more you know about agribusiness, the more skeptical you'll become that industry and government experts are watching out. It's clear that we are made no safer by monocultures of crops and animals, or by chemicals and toxins being pumped into our soil in the name of cheap food. True food security means diversifying food sources, making its production transparent, and ensuring that everyone has access to healthy, sustainable options. It is not building more walls around factory farms or moving all the animals inside. Surely it doesn't mean turning our farms into biohazard sites, where visitors must scrub down and don facility-issued clothing to gain access (if it's permitted at all).

Food shouldn't need to be irradiated to be safe. Animals shouldn't need to be pumped full of antibiotics. We shouldn't be ingesting food that is making us sick and depressed. We shouldn't be living on cocktails of drugs or weight-loss pills. Animals shouldn't be bred to grow so big so fast that their joints can't support their weight. And we shouldn't have people suffering from malnutrition in this land of plenty. The natural state of our body politic shouldn't be obese and passive. Obesity is intensely inconvenient, and physically and emotionally painful. It's also expensive. Estimates suggest that the direct costs of treating obesity-related conditions in the United States are $117 billion every year and headed higher, on a par with the amount we spend on fast food each year.

When you become aware of the realities of our current food system, it becomes harder to swallow other things as well: the indigestible lies, the government complicity, the junk culture. When you are connected to the land, directly or through farmers, you become a participant in the vital ground of this democracy. That's why we need to speak out against policies that allow industrial farms and other irresponsible entities to harm our well-being. Make your legislators aware of the issues and your concerns. They are accountable to you, and they are public servants—or at least should be.

It's also important to continue educating yourself (see the Resources section) and to express your concerns close to home and beyond. Read newspapers and journals, whether print or online, and if you feel moved, write letters to the editor raising concerns about factory farming and the importance of making compassionate eating choices. Join advocacy organizations. Distribute literature and share what you have learned with family, friends, and neighbors. Get involved with social groups and help organize community events. Be active in your place of worship or spiritual center, and let people know you care about how we eat and what happens to the animals. Be passionate and follow your heart, which will encourage and empower yourself and others. And listen to your gut. It is shocking what happens on factory farms; it is not wrong to feel that people should know about it and want it to stop.

Eating is a pleasure to be shared, and yet many of us have nothing but anxiety and guilt about it. Ultimately, how you decide to eat is your decision, but it should be clear from what I've described in this book that what you choose has real consequences for many individuals— literally billions of them. These are difficult topics, I know. When you talk about food and farming with anyone, you may step onto a cultural, political, familial, religious, and emotional battleground. We have very intense feelings about food, founded on myths and identities influenced by where and how we grew up, our agrarian roots, and an assumption that humans are different from other animals.

I recognize the strength of these beliefs. This is why, over the course of my activist life, I've always tried to be mindful of other perspectives, and through this to seek common ground. I believe it's important to act with compassion and respect. Even though I hold a vision of a vegan world and of agriculture free of the exploitation of animals, I am more than aware that this vision is unlikely to be achieved in my lifetime. This is why, although I am persistent, I am also patient. I have always thought it's better to do something positive and practical, and not to make the perfect an enemy of progress.

Over the years, I've seen many hopeful changes in the way society views animals, more than I anticipated when Farm Sanctuary began. There are more vegetarian and vegan restaurants in the United States than ever before. In academia, we're seeing the study of "animal sentience" and not just "animal science." Dozens of U.S. law schools are teaching courses on animal law, and increasingly bar associations have animal law committees. We are beginning to see a growing awareness, legal victories, and some progress on legislation. In addition, the media are beginning to pay attention to human-animal relationships and have even started to report on the once-hidden realities of factory farming. Those who care about animals can take heart and find in these little victories the sign of greater ones to come.

You're Invited

Consider this book an open invitation to visit us in New York or California. Getting to know the cows, pigs, chickens, sheep, goats, and other animals will revive you and maybe, as it has for many, transform you. If you can't come in person, why not "adopt" one of our animals? Farm Sanctuary has an Adopt-a-Farm Animal program whereby you can pay a monthly fee that helps care for the animals. You will receive a picture of the animal(s) you adopted along with updates about your animal(s), which you can share with others. (And if you think you can provide a home to two or more rescued farmed animals, please visit our website to find out more about our adoption program.) This Thanksgiving, instead of the traditional turkey dinner, why not adopt a turkey who lives at Farm Sanctuary? You don't need to invite a turkey to dinner the way we do, but you can celebrate the holiday with meatless Tofurky or Unturkey, both widely available in health food stores, in some supermarkets, or through the Internet.

Most people don't want to harm animals or tacitly accept cruelty. But I also know how hard it is to go up against a powerful system that offers you every opportunity to turn a blind eye to what happens to the animals. That's why I'm so moved by those within the industry who have risked their jobs and the scorn of their peers to stand up against abuse. They saw the animals and not the production units, and recognized that their treatment was unacceptable.

I once had a conversation with a filmmaker who told me about going to some built-up residential areas in Los Angeles. As he looked at those buildings with tier upon tier of identical apartments, he noticed wires snaking from the windows, each hooked up to a satellite dish. He saw the cables as intravenous drips, feeding the residents television's concoction of commercials and anesthetizing programming. I wondered to myself if we weren't more like the factory-farmed animals than we thought: all of us, locked in our cages, numbed by or pumped full of artificial stimulants, being fattened and sickened until we were ready to be taken away to our death.

When I walk around the Farm Sanctuary shelters, I look at the animals industrial agriculture has bred or treated with indignity, and marvel at their capacity to enjoy their lives, no matter how humble they may seem. They are not isolated. Some animals are kept apart from others because they're sick or, in a few cases, unable to get along with members of their own species. But there's always someone who's willing to tolerate their quirks and hang out with them. And they're always engaged in the world around them—sniffing the air, nuzzling the ground, rooting in the soil, pulling at the grass, pecking in the dirt, swimming in the pond, ruminating, or nesting. They are connected to the physical world in a way that we humans seem to have lost.

Isn't that what we need to do: reclaim our own animal natures after being production units for too long? To grasp the possibilities of being alive and empowered, rather than enslaved by old habits and assumptions as we sit and work in our individual cubicles? The animals show us the enjoyment of simple pleasures and of being in the moment. They teach us that we are of the world. And they tell us that, beneath the skin, we're all bodies together.

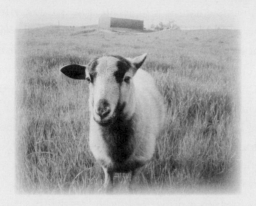

Persia

PROFILE: PERSIA

For reasons we won't ever know, Persia's mom—a Barbados sheep—rejected her, choosing to nurse only Persia's twin. Persia needed special care, including bottle feeding, to survive. But the farmer raising her didn't want to spend the time or money. Instead, he planned to send the days-old Persia to market, or simply let her die. A local animal control officer heard about Persia and offered to take her off the farmer's hands. He readily agreed, and she took the lamb home. While the officer and her daughter enjoyed Persia's company, they knew the lamb would be happier around other sheep, and Persia came to our Orland shelter.

Persia, whose coat is light beige and who has brownish wool on her face along with black stripes and black ears, made herself right at home. Many of the rescued animals are, at least initially, wary around people. Some are downright terrified. In contrast, Persia happily trotted up to everyone in range, bleating loudly and nibbling on people's fingers, right from the beginning. She was a popular lamb, to say the least. We named her after actress-musician Persia White, a good friend of Farm Sanctuary and farmed animals, as well as an environmentalist and advocate for human rights. Now a full-grown sheep, Persia is as popular as ever, and happy. She's become good friends with another once-orphaned sheep, Bleu, and the two of them can be found grazing, napping in piles of straw, and enjoying the rays of the California sun.

Epilogue: Finding Sanctuary

When Hilda died, we buried her in the garden at the Watkins Glen shelter, not far from the foundations of the barn built in the 1800s. In the spring, flowers form a blanket over the grave, and the herbs and other plants attract butterflies and bees. We etched a drawing of a lamb on the headstone along with this inscription: "Hilda, rescued from a stockyard, August 3, 1986, died of old age, September 25, 1997. Forever changing hearts and minds."

When we rescued Hilda and founded Farm Sanctuary, we had no idea that either would survive as long as they did, or touch so many. We simply wanted to get Hilda out of the stockyard. Ironically, Hilda probably did more to help others than anyone ever did for her. Thousands of visitors have been reconnected with farm life through Hilda (and the other animals) and, in doing so, reconnect with the finer aspects of their own humanity. At the sanctuary the animals can be who they are and people can allow themselves to care.

Twenty years later, we have rescued thousands of animals, have made hundreds of thousands of people aware of the plight of farmed animals, and have helped enact laws that will affect the lives of millions of them. Through the Watkins Glen and Orland sanctuaries, we have shown people that cows, pigs, chickens, turkeys, sheep, and all other farm animals are capable of awareness, feeling, and suffering—in some ways, suffering more intense than our own precisely because for most it never ends.

In the course of this work, the meaning of the word *sanctuary* has deepened for me. For every Hilda, Hope, or Cinci Freedom, we are aware that another creature—in just as much pain and just as deserving of care—is being denied a place of mercy. There are always more animals than we can provide shelter for. Even if we had space for five thousand, or five hundred thousand, or five million, or a thousand times that number, it wouldn't be enough. We'd still have to say, "Sorry, we can't take any more." So beyond providing a home for the animals we can take in, the sanctuaries act as a reminder that for billions of other farmed animals there is no respite or place of mercy.

The animals who do make it to our California and New York shelters embody the dangers of factory farming all too well. Because our society mainly eats the young, Farm Sanctuary is one of the few places in the country where it is possible to see the long-term effects of breeding for productivity and industrial confinement. As they age, the animals need additional care. Genetic alterations and the industry's standard practices have compromised their health in irreversible ways. So although looking after the animals is time-consuming, expensive, and sometimes emotionally painful, we feel responsible to provide the best care possible. By opening our hearts to the difficult and broken, a deeper healing can take place. That, for me, is the most profound of all the meanings of *sanctuary*.

And that's exactly what has happened. Over the years, many visitors to Farm Sanctuary weep when they see the condition of the animals and learn where they've come from. They cry for many reasons. Because they suddenly realize their food has a face. Because they discover how deeply they care about animals even if they've never put those feelings into words. Because they can finally relax with others who feel the way they do about animals. Because they think the problem is so immense that they cannot make a difference. Or because at least, and at last, the animals in front of them *are* free from crates, cages, and pens.

Many others, sometimes the same people, feel intensely happy and connected when they come to Farm Sanctuary. They revel in their time spent with animals most have never seen alive or up close before. And they get to do what so few of us ever do: see the animals doing what they do best—be themselves.

Our sanctuaries bear witness to the fact that we are responsible for everything that happens to these animals. That is work we accept, not only for the creatures in our care but also for people who come as guests. We honor their feelings of pain, empathy, and elation. By being a place where suffering and healing meet, where kindness has come out of cruelty, Farm Sanctuary is a place of wholeness.

*   *   *

In the future, I hope to open more sanctuaries, perhaps closer to cities so we can reach a larger population of people more easily. We also want to continue developing the Watkins Glen and Orland farms as places of refuge and transformation, for both animals and people. We'll continue to respond to animals in crisis and address systemic issues in the hope of stemming the flow of farmed animals in need of care. Many animal refuges are already full. As Bill McCoy of Lancaster Stockyards told me all those years ago, the monkey is still on our backs.

More farm animals are being cruelly treated and killed today than ever before, and agribusiness is doing all it can to make sure you don't know about it. I won't deny that it's an enormous wave of sorrow and suffering. It will strike some as wildly impractical even to try to turn back this tide. But as one friend who visited our sanctuary has written, "You can thank heaven for [that] kind of impracticality, for no great wrong has ever been overcome without it."

The vast scope of the problem is precisely why we cannot afford to stop. These issues touch us all, and each of us can make a difference every time we eat. Overcoming cruelty is something we can do one person, one choice, one act of conscience at a time. Eating meat is a habit we choose, not an unwritten law to be blindly obeyed. In the face of factory farming's harsh and violent spirit, every one of us has the power to say no and in doing so show the world that there is a kinder way.

When all the arguing is done, all the objections heard and excuses made, it comes down to this: if you're aware of something bad happening, are you going to try to make it better? We first saw Hilda and then many others lying on dead piles, took them home, and tried to make them well. We gave them a patch of earth on which to live. And then we tried to stop the conditions, attitudes, and assumptions that led to the dead pile in the first place.

At our best, we in the animal protection movement work to create change without resembling agribusiness in its arrogance and self-righteousness. We seek out abusers and ask that justice be done, but we recognize that not everyone in a bad business is a bad person. We attempt to prevent cruel practices without destroying the persons carrying them out ("love the sinner, hate the sin"). We recognize that sometimes people cause harm because they are uninformed, not evil. And every now and then, someone in the twisted world of industrial agriculture turns away in disgust and remorse. For farmers, too, there is a better way.

In efforts of generosity or love, it's common for those who offer help to feel repaid many times over by what they learn from the ones in need. Over the years, from the day we found Hilda stirring in the dead pile, the animals at Farm Sanctuary have taught me many things. They have made me thankful for what I have, real and authentic things. Animals have ways of their own, defined by directness and purity of intention, and none of us is so wise that we can't stand to learn a thing or two from their examples. Sometimes the animals at Farm Sanctuary simply remind me to get outside and revel in the sunshine.

Best of all, I have learned something about forgiveness. It's amazing to me that these creatures born into the cold and mechanized existence of factory farming, where the appearance of any human being only spelled more pain, could ever again bestow their trust, much less their friendship, on anyone of our species. Yet somehow they do, and it is a beautiful thing to see. If these farmed animals, after all that they have been through, can still learn to respect humanity, then surely we can learn to respect them.

In the evenings, when I walk out of my office in New York or California, I often pause to look out over the farm. In the pastures are the cows and goats and sheep. In their fields and mud holes are the pigs, the picture of contentedness. On the wind, I hear the roosters calling their hens. All of them, every night, are accounted for, all of them safe and protected. And each night, it is a gift to know that another day has passed that has in a small way made up for the time that billions of animals have spent in factory farms—far away, from here at least, from all the horror and all the hurt. It is the gift of a good life, granted to these survivors and returned in kind. I hope it will be your gift as well.

Appendix

Resources

There are many great sources for additional information on factory farming, farmed animals, animal welfare and rights, as well as places to research sustainable, humane food production, organic and local foods, and becoming vegetarian or vegan. New resources are emerging all the time, so it's impossible to include everything here. What follows are some websites, organizations, publications, and publishers I know of and that I encourage you to visit, learn more about, read, and contact.

WEBSITES TO HELP YOU FIND FARMERS' MARKETS, COMMUNITY-SUPPORTED AGRICULTURE PROGRAMS, AND VEGAN FOOD IN YOUR AREA

Local Harvest—www.localharvest.org
> Type in your zip code and find farmers' markets, family farms, food co-ops, and even community-supported agriculture (CSA) programs in your community or state.

HappyCow—www.happycow.net
> Global, searchable vegetarian dining guide and directory of natural health food stores, including nutrition and health tips, vegan recipes, raw foods, travel tips, and information on veganism and other vegetarian issues.

VegDining—www.vegdining.com
> Online guide to vegetarian restaurants around the world.

Veg for Life—www.VegForLife.org
> A Farm Sanctuary resource with how-tos, recipes, veg-friendly restaurant lists, and other information for people interested in cruelty-free living.

Alternative Farming Systems Information Center—www.nal.usda.gov/afsic/csa/
Site run by the USDA with resources on learning more about or locating CSAs.

There are local health food stores and food cooperatives in urban and rural communities throughout the United States, and they are a good source of organic and vegan food. Chains such as Whole Foods Market (www.wholefoodsmarket.com), Trader Joe's (www.traderjoes.com), Wild Oats (www.wildoats.com), and Earth Fare (www.earthfare.com) are good sources of healthy, sustainable foods, too. When shopping at these or other grocery stores, encourage them to offer more healthy, vegan foods.

FARM SANCTUARY WEB-BASED RESOURCES

www.FarmSanctuary.org
This is Farm Sanctuary's main website, which describes our various rescue, education, and advocacy efforts and provides opportunities for you to get involved.

www.AdoptATurkey.org
Provides resources for those interested in celebrating a new Thanksgiving tradition and saving a turkey rather than eating one. Includes vegetarian recipes, turkey industry facts, and holiday menu suggestions, along with selected turkeys that you can "adopt."

www.FarmAnimalShelters.org
Describes how to care for farm animals and operate a farm animal sanctuary. Links to shelters that care for rescued farm animals.

www.FactoryFarming.com
A wealth of information about the factory farming industry, including photos and videotape of intensive farming practices.

www.FarmSanctuaryKids.org
Provides information for grade-school-age youth to introduce them to farm animal issues in an age-appropriate way. Includes photos and educational activities for children, as well as resources for teachers.

www.NoDowners.org
Information about Farm Sanctuary's "No Downers" campaign to prevent the marketing and slaughter of animals too sick to stand, which includes details of current legislation and other advocacy efforts.

www.NoFoieGras.org

Website for Farm Sanctuary's "No Foie Gras" campaign. Includes information about current advocacy efforts, along with names of establishments that support or oppose the cruelty of foie gras, and what you can do to help.

www.NoVeal.org

Website for Farm Sanctuary's "No Veal" campaign. Includes information about current advocacy efforts, along with names of establishments that promote or oppose the cruelty of veal, and what you can do to help.

www.SentientBeings.org

Website for Farm Sanctuary's "Sentient Beings" campaign, which seeks to elevate the status of farm animals in the United States.

www.WalkForFarmAnimals.org

Information about getting active in Farm Sanctuary's annual autumn Walk for Farm Animals, which raises funds for and awareness of helping farm animals in communities across North America.

FARM SANCTUARY RESEARCH REPORTS

As of this writing, Farm Sanctuary has produced the following research reports. For a current list, please e-mail info@farmsanctuary.org or see www.farmsanctuary.org.

Farm Sanctuary, *Farm Animal Welfare: An Assessment of Product Labeling Claims, Industry Quality Assurance Guidelines, and Third Party Certification Standards.*

————, *Opinions of Veterinarians and Positions of the AVMA: Analysis of Eight Commonly Occurring Farming Practices.*

————, *Sentient Beings: A Summary of the Scientific Evidence Establishing Sentience in Farmed Animals.*

————, *U.S. Highway Accidents Involving Farm Animals.*

————, *The Welfare of Calves in Veal Production: A Summary of the Scientific Evidence.*

————, *The Welfare of Cattle in Beef Production: A Summary of the Scientific Evidence.*

————, *The Welfare of Cattle in Dairy Production: A Summary of the Scientific Evidence.*

————, *The Welfare of Ducks and Geese in Foie Gras Production: A Summary of the Scientific and Empirical Evidence.*

————, *The Welfare of Hens in Battery Cages: A Summary of the Scientific Evidence.*

————, *The Welfare of Sows in Gestation Crates: A Summary of the Scientific Evidence.*

————, *Unnatural Breeding Techniques and Results in Modern Turkey Production.*

Farm Sanctuary, *Unnatural Breeding Techniques and Results in Modern Dairy Production.*

Farm Sanctuary and Brighter Green, *The 2007 Farm Bill: A New Vision for U.S. Agriculture, Food Production, and Healthy Eating.*

ORGANIZATIONS

ANIMAL ADVOCACY ORGANIZATIONS

Animal Protection and Rescue League—www.aprl.org
Works to document and expose cruelty inflicted on animals and to protect their rights and habitats.

Animal Rights Foundation of Florida—www.animalrightsflorida.org
Raises awareness and advocates for animals throughout Florida, and played a key role in enacting the nation's first successful initiative to ban cruel factory-farming practice (i.e., gestation crates) in Florida in 2002.

Animal Rights International (ARI)—www.ari-online.org
Founded by Henry Spira and now headed by Peter Singer, ARI has placed ads and works to raise awareness about factory farming issues.

Animal Welfare Advocacy—www.animalwelfareadvocacy.org
The mission is to alleviate animal suffering and promote the well-being of animals through the legislative and political advocacy process.

Animal Welfare Institute (AWI)—www.awionline.org
A longtime presence in Washington, D.C., AWI lobbied to pass the Humane Slaughter Act in the 1950s, and today works with farmers to promote traditional farming practices.

Animals' Angels—www.animals-angels.de
An organization based in Germany that investigates and exposes the inhumane treatment of farm animals across Europe and around the globe.

Animal Legal Defense Fund—www.aldf.org
Works to protect the lives and advance the interests of animals through the legal system.

Association of Veterinarians for Animal Rights (AVAR)—www.avar.org
AVAR is an organization made up largely of veterinarians who are concerned about protecting animals from suffering.

Compassionate Consumers—www.compassionateconsumers.org

A not-for-profit animal advocacy organization focusing on preventing the cruel use of animals in agriculture.

Compassion in World Farming (CIWF)—www.ciwf.org.uk

Started by a farmer in Britain in the 1960s, CIWF has campaigned to eliminate the use of inhumane factory farming systems in Europe and elsewhere.

Compassion Over Killing (COK)—www.cok.net

COK works to end animal abuse by focusing on cruelty to animals in agriculture and promoting vegetarian eating.

DawnWatch—www.dawnwatch.com

Monitors media stories pertaining to animals and provides concerned citizens with suggestions for promoting animal-friendly reporting in print and broadcast.

Humane Society of the U.S. (HSUS)—www.humanesociety.org

With ten million members, this is the largest animal advocacy organization in the United States. It endeavors to protect all animals, including farmed animals.

Humane USA—www.humaneusa.org

The nation's leading political action committee dedicated to helping elect animal-friendly legislators.

Institute for Humane Education—www.humaneeducation.org

An educational organization dedicated to creating a humane world through humane education. Offers training for humane educators.

Jane Goodall Institute (JGI)—www.janegoodall.org

Founded by the famous primatologist, JGI asks individuals to take informed and compassionate actions to improve the environment of all living things.

Mercy for Animals—www.mercyforanimals.org

Dedicated to promoting nonviolence toward all sentient beings, through public education campaigns and demonstrations, undercover investigations, and open rescues.

People for the Ethical Treatment of Animals (PETA)—www.peta.org

Known for drawing attention to various forms of animal cruelty around the world, PETA promotes vegan living and urges reforms in the farming industry.

Roots and Shoots—www.rootsandshoots.org

A global network of more than eight thousand groups in almost a hundred countries through which youth undertake projects that promote care and concern for animals, the environment, and the human community.

United Poultry Concerns (UPC)—www.upc-online.org

Founded by Karen Davis, UPC focuses on relieving the exploitation and suffering of chickens and other domesticated birds.

VEGETARIAN AND VEGAN ORGANIZATIONS

American Vegan Society—www.americanvegan.org

Teaching a compassionate way of living, which includes veganism.

Christian Vegetarian Association—www.all-creatures.org/cva

Educates people about the health, environmental, and animal-related advantages of plant-based eating, and supports and encourages Christian vegetarians around the world.

Institute for Plant-Based Nutrition—www.plantbased.org

A group of plant-eaters and growers that educates the public about the benefits of plant-based nutrition.

International Vegetarian Union—www.ivu.org

International membership organization that works to promote vegetarianism throughout the world.

Jewish Vegetarians of North America—www.jewishveg.com

Advocates for vegetarianism from a Jewish perspective.

Meatout.org—www.meatout.org

On (or around) March 20, the first day of spring, thousands of people across the United States and around the world hold educational Meatout events to encourage people to forgo eating meat for at least one day, if not longer; coordinated by FARM, www.farmusa.org.

North American Vegetarian Society—www.navs-online.org

Dedicated to promoting the vegetarian way of life, and an organizer of annual vegetarian conferences.

Vegan Outreach—www.veganoutreach.org

Produces and distributes pamphlets and other literature that promote vegan living at colleges and universities throughout the United States.

Vegetarian Friends—www.vegetarianfriends.net

Provides inspiration and support for Quakers and other people of faith in the practice of love for animals and a vegetarian diet; publishes monthly journal, *The Peaceable Table*.

Vegetarian Resource Group—www.vrg.org

Dedicated to educating the public on vegetarianism and the interrelated issues of health, nutrition, ecology, ethics, and world hunger. Publishes *Vegetarian Journal,* which contains recipes and health information.

Vegsource.com—www.vegsource.com

Vegsource is an interactive online magazine with cutting-edge articles on a healthy diet and lifestyle, thousands of recipes, and book reviews, as well as numerous renowned doctors and other experts answering questions on active discussion boards.

VivaVegie Society—www.vivavegie.org

Undertakes vegetarian advocacy in New York City and also produces the popular pamphlet (now also a book), *101 Reasons Why I'm a Vegetarian.*

FOOD ADVOCACY AND
CONSUMER-ORIENTED ORGANIZATIONS

American Community Garden Association—www.communitygarden.org

Provides advice on starting a community garden, networking with community gardeners, and finding community gardens in your region.

Center for Food Safety—www.centerforfoodsafety.org

An organization established to challenge harmful food production technologies and promote sustainable alternatives.

Center for Science in the Public Interest—www.cspinet.org

Works to improve nutrition and health, food safety, alcohol policy, and share sound science; "Eating Green" program advocates for plant-based, ecologically friendly diets.

Consumers Union—www.consumersunion.org

An independent, nonprofit testing and information organization serving the interests of consumers.

Food and Water Watch—www.foodandwaterwatch.org

Works with grassroots organizations and other allies around the world to end corporate control of our food and water and create an economically and environmentally viable future.

Food Empowerment Project—www.foodispower.org

Seeks to create a more just and sustainable world by encouraging healthy food choices that reflect a more compassionate society by spotlighting the abuse of animals on farms, the depletion of natural resources, unfair working conditions for produce workers, and the unavailability of healthy foods in low-income areas.

Food Not Bombs—www.foodnotbombs.net

All-volunteer network that provides free, hot vegetarian meals and political support to low-income people in hundreds of communities in the Americas, Africa, Asia, the Middle East, Europe, and Australia.

Food Studies Institute—www.foodstudies.org

Promotes awareness of food, such as through Dr. Antonia Demas's groundbreaking curriculum, "Food Is Elementary," which aims to educate children about nutrition.

Just Food—www.justfood.org

Works to develop a just and sustainable food system in the New York City region.

Kitchens with Mission—www.kitchenswithmission.org

A food service training program for homeless people.

MadCowboy.com—www.madcowboy.com

Provides information about cattle rancher turned vegan advocate Howard Lyman, author of *Mad Cowboy*; mad cow disease; the dangers of current methods of food production; the values of a plant-based diet; and how every bite of food is a decision that affects all life on earth.

Organic Consumers Association—www.organicconsumers.org

Grassroots public-interest organization that represents the views and interests of U.S. organic food consumers.

Physicians Committee for Responsible Medicine (PCRM)—www.pcrm.org

Promotes preventive medicine, conducts clinical research, and encourages higher standards for ethics and effectiveness in research.

Safe Tables Our Priority (STOP)—www.safetables.org

Concerned about illnesses and loss of life caused by pathogens in food, Safe Tables Our Priority was formed to assist victims of food-borne illness, educate consumers, and advocate for policies that protect public health.

Vegan Organic Network—www.veganorganic.net

Provides information about vegan organic farming, which avoids animal by-products and uses vegetable compost, green manures, crop rotation, mulches, and other methods that are sustainable and ecologically viable.

Yale University Rudd Center for Food Policy and Obesity—www.yaleruddcenter
.org/home.aspx

Seeks to improve the world's diet, prevent obesity, and reduce weight stigma by
establishing connections between science and public policy, developing targeted
research, and encouraging frank dialogue among key constituents.

AGRICULTURE ADVOCACY AND
FAMILY-FARM-RELATED ORGANIZATIONS

Center for Rural Affairs—www.cfra.org

A private, nonprofit organization strengthening small businesses, family farms,
and rural communities.

Cornucopia Institute—www.cornucopia.org

An organization that fights for the family farming community, using research,
advocacy, and economic development strategies.

Farm Aid—www.farmaid.org

Works to keep family farmers on their land and bring together family farmers
and citizens to restore family-farm-centered agriculture.

Farmed Animal Net—www.farmedanimal.net

Directory of news and resources on farmed animal issues. Produces a weekly
e-news digest, available via e-mail. Sign up at the website.

Global Resource Action Center for the Environment (GRACE)—
www.factory farm.org

Works with communities to eliminate factory farming in favor of a sustainable
food production system that is healthful, economically viable, and ecologically
sound.

Government Accountability Project—www.whistleblower.org

Promotes government and corporate accountability by advancing occupational
free speech, defending whistle-blowers, and empowering citizen activists.

The Growing Connection—www.thegrowingconnection.org

Grassroots project developed by the Food and Agriculture Organization of
the United Nations (FAO) and the American Horticultural Society that links
people and cultures to introduce low-cost, water-efficient, and sustainable food-
growing innovations, hand in hand with wireless IT connectivity.

Institute for Agriculture and Trade Policy—www.iatp.org

Promotes resilient family farms, rural communities, and ecosystems around the world through research and education, science and technology, and advocacy.

Institute for Food and Development Policy/Food First—www.foodfirst.org

Works to shape how people think by analyzing the root causes of global hunger, poverty, and ecological degradation and developing solutions in partnership with movements working for social change.

Johns Hopkins University Center for a Livable Future—www.jhsph.edu/clf

Promotes research and develops and communicates information about the complex interrelationships among diet, food production, environment, and human health.

Leopold Center for Sustainable Agriculture—www.leopold.iastate.edu

Research and education center that works to develop sustainable agricultural practices that are both profitable and conserving of natural resources in Iowa and across the United States.

National Campaign for Sustainable Agriculture—www.sustainableagriculture.net

Nationwide partnership of individuals and organizations cultivating grassroots efforts to engage in policy development processes that result in food and agricultural systems and rural communities that are healthy, environmentally sound, profitable, humane, and just.

National Catholic Rural Life Conference—www.ncrlc.com

Membership organization grounded in a spiritual tradition that brings together the Church, care of community, and care of creation to work on a range of issues, among them food and agriculture and factory farming.

Northeast Organic Farmers Association (NOFA)—www.nofa.org

An organization of nearly four thousand farmers, gardeners, and consumers working to promote healthy food, organic farming practices, and a cleaner environment.

Oakland Institute—www.oaklandinstitute.org

Policy think tank working to increase public participation and promote fair debate on critical social, economic, and environmental issues in both national and international forums; works on food, agriculture, and trade issues.

Soil Association—www.soilassociation.org

UK-based organization championing sustainable, organic farming and human health.

Sustainable Agriculture Working Groups (organized regionally; search the web for specific regional websites)

A network of organizations working for a system of agriculture that is economically profitable, environmentally sound, family farm based, and socially just.

United Farm Workers of America (UFW)—www.ufw.org

Founded by César Chávez, UFW seeks to provide farm workers and other working people with the inspiration and tools to share in society's bounty.

ENVIRONMENTAL ORGANIZATIONS

Brighter Green—www.brightergreen.org

A public policy "action tank" working to advance public policy on the environment, animals, equity, and rights to ensure a future for all earth's inhabitants.

Center on Race, Poverty & the Environment (CRPE)—www.crpe-ej.org

A national environmental justice organization that provides legal and technical assistance to grassroots groups in low-income communities and communities of color fighting environmental hazards.

Circle of Life—www.circleoflife.org

Founded by Julia Butterfly Hill, works for peace, justice, and environmental sustainability and a transformation in the way humans interact with the earth and all living beings.

Climate Crisis Coalition—www.climatecrisiscoalition.org

Works to broaden the circle of individuals, organizations, and constituencies engaged in the global warming issue, to link it with other issues, and to provide a structure to forge a common agenda and advance action plans with a united front.

Earth Island Institute—www.earthisland.org

Develops and supports education and activism that counteract threats to the biological and cultural diversity that sustain the environment.

Earthjustice—www.earthjustice.org

Protects people, wildlife, and natural resources by providing free legal representation to citizen groups to enforce environmental laws in the United States.

Environmental Working Group (EWG)—www.ewg.org

EWG has been conducting environmental investigations since 1993; tracks federal farm subsidies.

Greenpeace—www.greenpeace.org

Campaigns using education and peaceful direct action to address a number of environmental issues, including global warming, deforestation, ocean destruction, whaling, and nuclear weapons and power.

Natural Resources Defense Council (NRDC)—www.nrdc.org

Aims to safeguard the earth, its people, plants, and animals, and the natural systems on which all life depends; works on factory farm issues.

Sierra Club—www.sierraclub.org

The oldest and largest grassroots environmental organization in the United States; works on factory farm issues.

Union of Concerned Scientists—www.ucsusa.org

An independent, nonprofit alliance of more than a hundred thousand concerned citizens and scientists.

Waterkeeper Alliance—www.waterkeeper.org

Headed by Robert F. Kennedy Jr.; works to promote water conservation and healthy waterways throughout the United States; has a program on factory farms.

World Rainforest Information Portal—www.rainforestweb.org

Gateway for global information and resources about threats to rainforests worldwide and campaigns to stop the destruction.

Worldwatch Institute—www.worldwatch.org

Policy think tank focused on the transition to an environmentally sustainable and socially just society; research includes factory farming and sustainable agriculture.

MAGAZINES AND PUBLISHERS

Animals' Voice—www.animalsvoice.com

Independent, networking source of information, news, campaigns, boycotts, action alerts, editorials, and photography about animal rights and its defenders. Print and online editions.

Book Publishing Company—www.thefarm.org/businesses/bpc.html

Offers books on how to create a more sustainable and healthful way of life. Publishes many vegetarian cookbooks.

E Magazine—www.emagazine.com

A bimonthly clearinghouse of information, news, and resources for people concerned about the environment who want to know what they can do to make a difference.

Herbivore—www.herbivoremagazine.com

Magazine featuring music, arts, politics, and contemporary culture from a vegan perspective.

Lantern Books—www.lanternbooks.com

Publisher of books on vegetarianism, animal advocacy, environmentalism, spirituality, and social justice.

Veg News—www.vegnews.com

The leading magazine on the vegetarian lifestyle; features lifestyle tips, products, recipes, and news.

Vegetarian Times—www.vegetariantimes.com

Provides a variety of vegetarian and vegan recipes, as well as cooking tips, entertaining suggestions, and health advice.

BOOKS (in addition to those included in References)

ANIMAL AWARENESS

Balcombe, Jonathon. *Pleasurable Kingdom: Animals and the Nature of Feeling Good.* New York: Macmillan, 2006.

Bauston, Gene. *Battered Birds, Crated Herds: How We Treat the Animals We Eat.* Watkins Glen, N.Y.: Farm Sanctuary, Inc., 1996.

Davis, Karen. *More Than a Meal: The Turkey in History, Myth, Ritual, and Reality.* New York: Lantern Books, 2001.

———. *Prisoned Chickens, Poisoned Eggs: An Inside Look at the Modern Poultry Industry.* Summertown, Tenn.: Book Publishing Company, 1996.

Mason, Jim. *An Unnatural Order: Why We Are Destroying the Planet and Each Other.* New York: Lantern Books, 2005.

Mason, Jim, and Peter Singer. *Animal Factories.* New York: Three Rivers Press, 1990.

Masson, Jeffrey Moussaieff. *The Pig Who Sang to the Moon: The Emotional World of Farm Animals.* New York: Ballantine Books, 2003.

Masson, Jeffrey Moussaieff, with Susan McCarthy. *When Elephants Weep: The Emotional Lives of Animals.* New York: Delta, 1996.

Newkirk, Ingrid. *Making Kind Choices: Everyday Ways to Enhance Your Life Through Earth- and Animal-Friendly Living.* New York: St. Martin's Press, 2005.

Regan, Tom. *Empty Cages: Facing the Challenge of Animal Rights.* Lanham, Md.: Rowman and Littlefield, 2004.

Rifkin, Jeremy. *Beyond Beef: The Rise and Fall of the Cattle Culture.* New York: Dutton, 1992.

Rowe, Martin. *The Way of Compassion: Vegetarianism, Environmentalism, Animal Advocacy, and Social Justice.* New York: Stealth Technologies, 1999.

Scully, Matthew. *Dominion: The Power of Men, the Suffering of Animals, and the Call to Mercy.* New York: St. Martin's Press, 2003.

Singer, Peter. *Animal Liberation.* New York: Harper Perennial, 2001.

———, ed. *In Defense of Animals: The Second Wave.* Boston: Blackwell, 2005.

Wolfson, David J. *Beyond the Law: Agribusiness and the Systemic Abuse of Animals Raised for Food or Food Production.* Watkins Glen, N.Y.: Farm Sanctuary, Inc., 1999.

COOKBOOKS

Atchison, Jeani-Rose. *Everyday Vegan: 300 Recipes for Healthful Living.* Berkeley, Calif.: North Atlantic Books, 2002.

Barnard, Tanya, and Sarah Kramer. *How It All Vegan! Irresistible Recipes for an Animal-Free Diet.* Vancouver, B.C.: Arsenal Pulp Press, 2000.

Davis, Brenda, and Vesanto, Melina. *Becoming Vegan: A Complete Guide to Adopting a Healthy Plant-Based Diet.* Summertown, Tenn.: Book Publishing Company, 2000.

Gartenstein, Devra. *The Accidental Vegan.* Berkeley, Calif.: Ten Speed Press, 2000.

Hagler, Louise, and Dorothy R. Bates. *The New Farm Vegetarian Cookbook.* Summertown, Tenn.: Book Publishing Company, 1988.

McCarthy, Brian. *The Vegan Family Cookbook.* New York: Lantern Books, 2005.

Moskowitz, Isa Chandra. *Vegan with a Vengeance.* New York: Marlowe and Company, 2005.

Petrovna, Tanya. *The Native Foods Restaurant Cookbook.* Boston, Mass.: Shambhala Publications, Inc., 2003.

Pierson, Joy, and Bart Potenza, with Barbara Scott-Goodman. *The Candle Café Cookbook: More Than 150 Enlightened Recipes from New York's Renowned Vegan Restaurant.* New York: Clarkson Potter Publishers, 2003.

Robertson, Robin. *Vegan Planet.* Boston: Harvard Common Press, 2003.

Stepaniak, Joanne. *The Ultimate Uncheese Cookbook.* Summertown, Tenn.: Book Publishing Company, 2003.

———. *Vegan Vittles: Recipes Inspired by the Critters of Farm Sanctuary.* Summertown, Tenn.: Book Publishing Company, 1996.

———. *Vegan Vittles: Second Helpings: Down-Home Cooking for Everyone.* Summertown, Tenn.: Book Publishing Company, 2007.

Wasserman, Debra. *Simply Vegan.* 3rd ed. Baltimore: Vegetarian Resource Group, 1999.

HEALTH, FARMING, AND FOOD ISSUES

Adams, Carol. *Living Among Meat Eaters.* New York: Continuum, 2003.

Barnard, Neal. *Food for Life.* New York: Three Rivers Press, 1993.

Campbell, T. Colin. *The China Study: The Most Comprehensive Study of Nutrition Ever Conducted and the Startling Implications for Diet, Weight Loss, and Long-term Health.* Dallas, Tex.: BenBella Books, 2006 (www.thechinastudy.com).

Demas, Antonia. *Food Is Elementary: A Hands-on Curriculum for Young Students.* Trumansburg, N.Y.: Food Studies Institute, 2001.

Esselstyn, Caldwell. *Prevent and Reverse Heart Disease.* New York: Avery, 2007.

Goodall, Jane. *Harvest for Hope: A Guide to Mindful Eating.* New York: Warner Books, 2005.

Halweil, Brian. *Eat Here: Reclaiming Homegrown Pleasures in a Global Supermarket.* New York: W. W. Norton, 2004.

Imhoff, Daniel. *Food Fight: The Citizen's Guide to a Food and Farm Bill.* Healdsburg, Calif.: Watershed Media, 2007.

Lappé, Anna, and Bryant Terry. *Grub: Ideas for an Urban Organic Kitchen.* New York: Tarcher, 2006.

Lovenheim, Peter. *Portrait of a Burger as a Young Calf: The Story of One Man, Two Cows, and the Feeding of a Nation.* New York: Harmony Books, 2002.

Lyman, Howard. *Mad Cowboy.* New York: Scribner, 1998.

Marcus, Erik. *Vegan: The New Ethics of Eating.* Ithaca, N.Y.: McBooks Press, 1998.

McDougall, John, and Mary McDougall. *The McDougall Program for a Healthy Heart: A Life-Saving Approach to Preventing and Treating Heart Disease.* New York: Plume, 1998.

Midkiff, Ken. *The Meat You Eat: How Corporate Farming Has Endangered America's Food Supply.* New York: St. Martin's Press, 2004.

Nestle, Marion. *Food Politics: How the Food Industry Influences Nutrition and Health.* Berkeley: University of California Press, 2003.

———. *What to Eat: An Aisle by Aisle Guide to Savvy Food Choices and Good Eating.* New York: North Point Press, 2006.

Ornish, Dean. *Dr. Dean Ornish's Program for Reversing Heart Disease: The Only System Scientifically Proven to Reverse Heart Disease Without Drugs or Surgery.* Rev. ed. New York: Ballantine Books, 2008.

Rice, Pamela. *101 Reasons Why I'm a Vegetarian.* New York: Lantern Books, 2005.

Robbins, John. *Diet for a New America.* Walpole, N.H.: Stillpoint Publishing, 1987.

———. *The Food Revolution.* York Beach, Maine: Conari Press, 2001.

Saunders, Kerrie. *The Vegan Diet as Chronic Disease Prevention: Evidence Supporting the New Four Food Groups.* New York: Lantern Books, 2003.

Singer, Peter, and Jim Mason. *The Way We Eat: Why Our Food Choices Matter.* New York: Rodale, 2006.

Spurlock, Morgan. *Don't Eat This Book: Fast Food and the Supersizing of America.* New York: Putnam, 2005.

Stepaniak, Joanne. *Being Vegan: Living with Conscience, Conviction, and Compassion.* Lincolnwood, Ill.: Lowell House, 2000.

Tuttle, Will. *The World Peace Diet.* New York: Lantern Books, 2005.

WHERE TO SHOP FOR VEGAN ITEMS

Alternative Outfitters—www.alternativeoutfitters.com

Carries a collection of vegan shoes, handbags, accessories, and cruelty-free personal care items.

Ethical Wares (UK)—www.ethicalwares.com

Mail order company that supplies vegan shoes, fair trade products, and accessories for a cruelty-free lifestyle; it even has a music collection.

Farm Sanctuary—www.farmsanctuary.org

In addition to operating gift shops at our shelters, Farm Sanctuary sells a variety of shirts, cards, books, and other items through our website.

Herbivore—www.herbivoreclothing.com

Offers clothes, cards, art, and other accessories to support vegan living.

Moo Shoes—www.mooshoes.com

New York City–based company that sells women's shoes, men's shoes, casual shoes, and both chic and formal shoes, as well as belts, wallets, jackets, and other accessories without any animal by-products.

Pangea—www.veganstore.com

Offers vegan shoes, belts, jackets, foods, body care, T-shirts, wallets, vitamins, cosmetics, gift baskets, chocolates, candles, books, and more.

Vegan Essentials—www.veganessentials.com

Offers a wide range of vegan products, from clothing to household items, food, and personal care products.

Vegan Unlimited—www.veganunlimited.com

Sells various vegan products, including clothes and cosmetics, food, and gift baskets.

Vegetarian Shoes (UK)—www.vegetarian-shoes.co.uk

Provides a wide range of non-leather shoes and other accessories.

REFERENCES

In addition to the citations noted for each chapter, the information in this book was developed over the past twenty years through communicating variously with agribusiness workers and executives, academics, and government officials; reviewing numerous industry journals and trade publications; observing conditions firsthand during visits to hundreds of farms, stockyards, and slaughterhouses across the United States; caring for chickens, pigs, cows, turkeys, sheep, and other animals rescued from abuse; and producing Farm Sanctuary research reports and comments on various aspects of the animal farming industries. Farm Sanctuary's research reports, which are listed in the Resources section on pages 235-36, are reviewed and updated periodically.

Eisnitz, Gail A. *Slaughterhouse: The Shocking Story of Greed, Neglect, and Inhumane Treatment Inside the U.S. Meat Industry.* Amherst, N.Y.: Prometheus Books, 1997.

Grandin, Temple, and Catherine Johnson. *Animals in Translation: Using the Mysteries of Autism to Decode Animal Behavior.* New York: Scribner, 2004.

Greger, Michael. *Bird Flu: A Virus of Our Own Hatching.* New York: Lantern Books, 2006.

Midkiff, Ken. *The Meat You Eat: How Corporate Farming Has Endangered America's Food Supply.* New York: St. Martin's Press, 2004.

Nierenberg, Danielle. *Happier Meals: Rethinking the Global Meat Industry.* Washington, D.C.: Worldwatch Institute, 2005.

Patterson, Charles. *Eternal Treblinka: Our Treatment of Animals and the Holocaust.* New York: Lantern Books, 2002.

Pollan, Michael. *The Omnivore's Dilemma: A Natural History of Four Meals.* New York: Penguin, 2006.

Schlosser, Eric. *Fast Food Nation: The Dark Side of the All-American Meal.* New York: HarperCollins Perennial, 2002.

Singer, Peter. *Ethics into Action: Henry Spira and the Animal Rights Movement.* Lanham, Md.: Rowman and Littlefield, 1998.

Striffler, Steve. *Chicken: The Dangerous Transformation of America's Favorite Food.* New Haven, Conn.: Yale University Press, 2005.

Stull, Donald D., Michael J. Broadway, and David Griffith. *Any Way You Cut It: Meat Processing and Small-Town America.* Lawrence: University of Kansas Press, 2000.

Sunstein, Cass, and Martha Nussbaum, eds. *Animal Rights: Current Debates and New Directions.* New York: Oxford University Press, 2004.

Notes

CHAPTER ONE: THE ROAD TO LANCASTER

8 *It was the beef industry that pioneered industrial farming:* See Schlosser, 137.

8 *By 1900, four hundred million animals had been slaughtered:* James R. Barrett, *Work and Community in the Jungle: Chicago's Packinghouse Workers, 1894–1922* (Urbana: University of Illinois Press, 1987), 15, 19, quoted in Patterson, 58.

8 *Inside the slaughterhouses, workers turned live animals into meat:* See Patterson, 72ff.

9 *Presented with these abuses, the Federal Trade Commission:* See Schlosser, 137.

10 *One postwar innovation in chemistry was chemical fertilizer:* See Pollan, 41.

10 *The call went out from Ezra Taft Benson:* See Midkiff, 2. This mantra was also echoed by Earl Butz, Richard Nixon's second secretary of agriculture. See Pollan, 52.

10 Pig, beef, dairy, and poultry farm information from 1950s to 2005: USDA, National Agricultural Statistics Service, *Agricultural Statistics 2006,* published by the U.S. Government Printing Office, Washington, D.C., 2006 (www .usda.gov/nass).

11 *an extraordinary 90* billion *eggs in 2005:* Donald Bell, "The U.S. Poultry Industry: Production and Values 2005," An Egg Economics Update, University of California, Riverside, June 2006 (http://animalscience.ucdavis.edu/avian/ eeu706.pdf, viewed August 2006).

11 *one in four people in the U.S. lived on a farm:* See Pollan, 34.

11 *only 0.7 percent of the U.S. population:* See Midkiff, 2.

11 *we see arranged on our supermarket shelves:* See Pollan, 100–8, for the consequences of overproduction.

12 Figures for revenues for ConAgra, Smithfield, Cargill, and Tyson come from www.conagra.com, www.smithfieldfood.com, www.cargill.com, and www .tyson.com/Corporate (all viewed August 2006).

12 *the top four cattle processors:* See Michael Stumo, "In Firm Control: Industrial Concentration in the U.S. Livestock Market," *Multinational Monitor,* July/August 2000.

12 *In 1950, just over 1 billion farmed animals:* See USDA, National Agricultural Statistics Service, *Agricultural Statistics 2006.*

CHAPTER TWO: SAVING HILDA

20 *Lancaster Stockyards was one of the oldest in the United States:* Jack Brubaker, "Lancaster Stockyards, Once the Largest East of Chicago, Hangs in There," *Lancaster Intelligencer Journal,* November 13, 1995.

21 *Lancaster was still handling over 300,000 animals a year:* Kimberley Jones, "Group Is 'Big Brother' to Farm Animals," *York Sunday News,* May 29, 1988.

31 *"I'm not jubilant about having to file cruelty charges":* Daina Savage, "Cruelty Citation Splits Animal Rights Group, Lancaster Stockyards," *Lancaster Intelligencer Journal,* October 14, 1992.

33 *"If we decide to make a big deal of this":* Daina Savage, "Lancaster Stockyards Found Guilty of Cruelty to Animals," *Lancaster Intelligencer Journal,* April 29, 1993.

34 *Later, McCoy himself acknowledged: The Farmer,* April 20, 1991.

34 *"Lancaster Stockyards, Once the Largest East of Chicago":* Jack Brubaker, "Lancaster Stockyards, Once the Largest East of Chicago, Hangs in There," *Lancaster Intelligencer Journal,* November 13, 1995.

35 *In April 2006, almost two decades:* Tim Mekeel, "Stockyard Deal: Developer of Target Mall Plans Mix of Stores, Offices, Housing," *Lancaster New Era,* April 12, 2006.

CHAPTER THREE: MAD COWS AND WASHINGTON

43 *"If I went by mail":* Library of Congress, "H. Con. Res. 175, Expressing the sense of Congress that the Humane Methods of Slaughter Act of 1958 should be fully enforced so as to prevent needless suffering of animals," 107th Congress of the United States, June 2001.

44 *The P&SA sent a letter:* Letter to stockyard owners and operators from Virgil Rosendale, administrator of the USDA's Packers and Stockyards Administration, July 8, 1991.

45 Examples from GIPSA reports on downed cows: United States Department of Agriculture before the Secretary of Agriculture re Amarillo Livestock Auction, Inc.; P.&S. Docket No. D-92-65, April 30, 1992. United States Department of Agriculture before the Secretary of Agriculture re Crockett Livestock Sales Company, Inc. and Danny W. Cobb; P.&S. Docket No. D-93-74, July 8, 1994.

45 *GIPSA appealed the ruling:* United States Department of Agriculture before the Secretary of Agriculture re Arizona Livestock Auction, Inc.; P.&S. Docket No. D-96-26; Order Denying Petition for Reconsideration, January 13, 1997.

46 *In 1986, Britain identified the first case of mad cow disease:* "BSE Inquiry—The Final Stage, Chronology of Events," BBC News (www.bbc.co.uk, viewed July 2006).

46 *Three people in the United Kingdom died of vCJD in 1995:* See "BSE Inquiry—The Final Stage, Chronology of Events."

46 *In 1993, despite the U.S. government's assurances:* "Transmissible Spongiform Encephalopathies—Impacts on Animal and Human Health," *Developments in Biological Standardization* 80 (1993): 111–18; R. F. Marsh and R. A. Bessen, *Epidemiologic and Experimental Studies on Transmissible Mink Encephalopathy.*

47 *In other words, they became downed cows:* J. R. Cutlip et al., "Intracerebral Transmission of Scrapie to Cattle," *Journal of Infectious Diseases* 169 (1994): 814–20.

47 *Nobody keeps track or knows the number:* USDA, Animal and Plant Health Inspection Service (APHIS), "Bovine Spongiform Encephalopathy (BSE)," May 20, 2004.

47 Excerpts from USDA response to Farm Sanctuary: Letter to Farm Sanctuary denying a petition to prohibit the slaughter of downed animals from Daniel L. Engeljohn, Ph.D., Director, Regulations Development and Analysis Division, Office of Policy, Program Development and Evaluation, USDA, Food Safety and Inspection Service (FSIS), Washington, D.C., March 25, 1999.

49 *"As I stand here before you":* Gary Ackerman (U.S. Representative), Farm Security Act of 2001, House of Representatives, October 4, 2001 (see http://thomas. loc.gov/cgi-bin/query/F?r107:1:./temp/~r107IEvmPc:e213139, viewed August 2006).

50 *Soon, however, evidence of a danger:* USDA, FSIS, "Bovine Spongiform Encephalopathy—Mad Cow Disease," Fact Sheets, March 2005 (www.fsis .usda.gov, viewed August 2006).

51 *Six days later, on December 30:* USDA, FSIS, "Bovine Spongiform Encephalopathy—Mad Cow Disease," Fact Sheets.

51 *Alarmingly, a 2006 report:* Office of Inspector General, "Audit Report: Animal and Plant Health Inspection Service (Bovine Spongiform Encephalopathy (BSE) Surveillance Program—Phase II and Food Safety Inspection Service Controls Over BSE Sampling, Specified Risk Materials, and Advanced Meat Recovery Products—Phase III. USDA," Report No. 50601-10-KC, January 2006 (see www.nodowners.org/USDA_2006.pdf, viewed August 2006).

51 *Whatever the reason for not testing all:* Steve Stecklow, "U.S. Falls Behind in Tracking Cattle to Control Disease," *Wall Street Journal,* June 21, 2006.

52 *Under the new policy:* "U.S. to Reduce Mad Cow Testing After Few Cases Found (Update 2)," Bloomberg, July 20, 2006 (www.bloomberg.com, viewed August 2006).

52 *When the Kansas-based beef processor:* Pete Hisey, "Creekstone Sues USDA over BSE Testing," Meatingplace.com, March 24, 2006 (www.Meatingplace.com, viewed August 2006).

CHAPTER FIVE: CALIFORNIA, HERE WE COME

71 *the state is also number one:* California Department of Food and Agriculture, California Agricultural Resource Directory 2005 (see www.cdfa.ca.gov, viewed August 2006).

72 *California is also the nation's top producer:* USDA, cited in California Dairy Quality Assurance Program, "Dairy Industry Facts" (see www.cdqa.org, viewed July 2006).

79 *While many of the approximately six million sheep:* USDA, "Livestock, Dairy and Poultry Outlook," January 2006 (see www.ers.usda.gov, viewed August 2006).

79 *Approximately four to five million lambs:* USDA, National Agricultural Statistics Service (NASS), Agricultural Statistics Board, "All Sheep and Lamb Inventory Shows Slight Decrease," July 21, 2006 (see http://usda.mannlib. cornell.edu/usda/current/SheeGoat/SheeGoat-07-21-2006.pdf, viewed August 2006).

CHAPTER SIX: WHAT'S WRONG WITH THE FACTORY FARM TODAY

84 *the roughly six million breeding sows:* A. B. Lawrence and E.M.C. Terlouw, "A Review of Behavioral Factors Involved in the Development and Continued Performance of Stereotypic Behavior in Pigs," *Journal of Animal Science* 71 (1993): 2815–25. See also Farm Sanctuary, *The Welfare of Sows in Gestation Crates: A Summary of the Scientific Evidence.*

87 *Federal subsidies or farm aid totaled $25 billion in 2005:* Dan Morgan et al., "Farm Program Pays $1.3 Billion to People Who Don't Farm," *Washington Post,* July 2, 2006.

87 *According to a 2006 report prepared by the Environmental Working Group:* EWG, "$1.5 Billion Bonus Subsidy in Emergency Spending Bill Is Unfair, Wasteful Response to Agriculture's Increased Energy Costs" (see www.ewg .org/reports/agsupp2006, viewed August 2006).

87 *The federal government also continues to provide subsidies:* See Midkiff, 54–55. Also the National Resources Conservation Service's Environmental Quality Incentives Program and www.wa.nrcs.usda.gov/programs/eqip/FY06/index .html, viewed August 2006.

87 *According to the Institute for Agriculture and Trade Policy (IATP):* IATP, "Below-Cost Feed Crops: An Indirect Subsidy for Industrial Animal Factories," June 2006 (www.itap.org, viewed August 2006).

88 *Large slaughterhouses that kill cattle:* "Dry as a Bone," *Drovers,* July 15, 2006. See also *Food Systems Insider,* July 6, 2006.

89 *In 2005, for instance, each American ate a record high amount:* John Lawrence, "Long Term Meat Production and Consumption Trends," *Iowa Farm Outlook,* February 2006 (www.thepoultrysite.com/FeaturedArticle/fatopic.asp? AREA=FeaturedArticle&Display=527, viewed August 2006).

89 *Currently, 64.5 percent of U.S. adults:* U.S. Centers for Disease Control and Prevention data, cited in American Obesity Association, "Obesity in the U.S." (see www.obesity.org, viewed July 2006).

89 *Globally, the World Health Organization:* Overweight statistic from WHO, "Obesity and Overweight, Facts" (www.who.int, viewed August 2006).

89 Hunger statistic: Food and Agriculture Organization of the United Nations (FAO), *State of Food Insecurity in the World 2005* (ftp://ftp.fao.org/docrep/fao/008/a0200e/a0200e00.pdf, viewed August 2006).

89 *This has resulted in agribusiness:* See Midkiff, 12. Also see Margaret Mellon, "Hogging It: Estimates of Antimicrobial Abuse in Livestock," Union of Concerned Scientists' Food and Environment Program January 2001; and statement by coauthor Margaret Mellon on the report's release. (see www.ucsusa.org/food_and_environment/antibiotics_and_food/margaret-mellon-on-hogging-it.html, viewed August 2006).

89 *Then there are mad cow disease:* Mark Winnie, "Meat-Industrial Complex: How Factory Farms Undercut Public Health," *In These Times*, March 22, 2006. Also Natural Resources Defense Council, "Pollution from Giant Livestock Farms Threatens Public Health" (see www.nrdc.org, viewed August 2006). Also Steven R. Kirkhorn, "Community and Environmental Health Effects of Concentrated Animal Feeding Operations," *Minnesota Medicine*, 2002, cited in Nierenberg, 30–32.

89 *social sicknesses:* See Schlosser, 83–87. For the problems with alcohol and spousal abuse, see Eisnitz, 87–88, and Stull, Broadway, and Griffith. *"can also expect to be confronted with school overcrowding, homelessness, housing shortages, elevated unemployment, crime, and social disorders":* See Stull, Broadway, and Griffith, 4.

91 *Tyson is so big:* See Striffler, 53–54.

91 *Brian Halweil of the Worldwatch Institute:* Brian Halweil, "Where Have All the Farmers Gone?" *World Watch*, September/October 2000.

92 *It is also perhaps why the suicide rate:* See Schlosser, 146.

93 *In 2001 foot-and-mouth disease:* "Beginnings of a Crisis," BBC News, July 22, 2002, and Martin Cassidy, "Living Through Foot and Mouth Crisis," BBC News, December 25, 2001 (see www.bbc.co.uk, viewed August 2006).

93 *When President Lincoln established:* USDA, National Agricultural Library, "Abraham Lincoln and Agriculture" (see www.nal.usda.gov, viewed July 2006).

CHAPTER SEVEN: THE REAL DEAL ON VEAL

100 *Pallor and tenderness:* Farm Sanctuary, *The Welfare of Calves in Veal Production: A Summary of the Scientific Evidence.* See also American Veal Association, "The Veal Story."

102 *Since the launch of the no-veal campaign:* USDA, April 14, 2004, "Livestock, Dairy, and Poultry Outlook" (see www.ers.usda.gov/Publications/LDP/apr04/ldpm118t.pdf#search=%22veal%20consumption%20down%22, viewed August 2006).

104 *In research conducted at Texas A&M University:* T. H. Friend and G. R. Dellmeier, "Common Practices and Problems Related to Artificially Rearing Calves: An Ethological Analysis," *Applied Animal Behavior Science* 20 (1988): 47–62.

104 *A wealth of studies:* European Commission, Animal Health and Welfare, "Animal Welfare on the Farm: Calves" (see http://ec.europa.eu/food/animal/welfare/farm/calves_en.htm, viewed August 2006).

104 *Each year, about seven hundred thousand male calves:* "The American Veal Industry: Producing a Special Product" (see www.vealfarm.com/edu-resources/downloads/special-product.pdf, viewed August 2006).

104 *Industry representatives have even suggested:* New Jersey General Assembly Environment and Solid Waste Meeting, N.J. Office of Legislative Services, Thursday, January 16, 2003.

105 *a spokesman for the American Veal Association:* Elizabeth Weise, "Growth Hormones in Veal Spark Debate," *USA Today,* April 1, 2004.

CHAPTER EIGHT: HOW NOW MILK COW?

114 *The sixteen hundred dairies in California's Central Valley:* Natural Resources Defense Council, "America's Animal Factories: How States Fail to Prevent Pollution from Livestock Waste. California" (see www.nrdc.org/water/pollution/factor/stcal.asp, "Top 50 Cities in the U.S. by Population and Rank," www.infoplease.com/ipa/A0763098.html, and World City Populations, www.pubquizhelp.34sp.com/geo/popcity.html, all viewed August 2006).

114 *Each cow produces 120 pounds of wet manure:* See www.epa.gov/region09/animalwaste/problem.html, viewed August 11, 2007.

114 *these huge operations are prone to outbreaks:* Jan Suszkiw, "Agricultural Research Service, New Anti-Mastitis Weapon on Tap for Dairy Cows," USDA, February 13, 2006 (see www.ars.usda.gov/is/pr/2006/060213.htm, viewed August 2006). Also A. C. Fitzgerald and M. L. Looper, "Non-Antibiotic Treatment of Postpartum Dairy Cows with Fever and Metabolic Disorders," *Professional Animal Scientist* 1, 2 (2003) (see http://findarticles.com/p/articles/mi_qa4035/is_200312/ai_n9319320, viewed August 2006). Also USDA, Agricultural Research Service, "Improving Milk Quality by Reducing Mastitis in Dairy Cattle," Annual Report 2003 (see www.ars.usda.gov/research/projects/projects.htm?ACCN_NO=404906&showpars=true&fy=2003, viewed August 2006).

115 *Because California's population:* U.S. Census Bureau, Population Pyramids of California (see www.census.gov/population/projections/05PyrmdCA3.pdf, viewed September 2006).

115 *in the heat wave that hit California:* Figures drawn from various news reports: "California Heat Wave Kills 25,000 Cattle: Official," *Agence France-Presse,* July 27, 2006; Dennis Pollock with Robert Rodriguez, "Record Heat Is Cow Killer," *Fresno Bee,* July 26, 2006; John Holland, "Dairy Industry Claims $1B Loss as Cows Die," *Modesto Bee,* July 29, 2006; Jennifer Steinhauer, "Unrelenting California Heat Wave Is Blamed for More than 100 Deaths," *New York Times,* July 28, 2006; and "California Heat Wave Death Toll Tops 130," Associated Press, July 28, 2006.

115 Ferreira quote: Lynda Geldhill, "Dairy Cows Dying: Many Ripening Crops at Risk," *San Francisco Chronicle,* July 26, 2006.

116 one-third of all dairy cattle in all fifty U.S. states have been injected with the hormone: See Monsanto spokesman quoted in Stephen J. Hedges, "Monsanto Having a Cow in Milk Label Dispute," *Chicago Tribune,* April 15, 2007.

116 *According to Canadian researchers:* D. S. Kronfeld, "Recombinant Bovine Somatotropin and Animal Welfare." *Journal of the American Veterinary Medicine Association* 216 (2000): 1719–22.

117 *While only 3.5 percent of dairy products:* Statistics cited in Steve Karnowski, "Organic Dairy Growth Raises Concerns," Associated Press, June 27, 2006.

117 *Some of these farms:* Karnowski, "Organic Dairy Growth."

117 *The Organic Consumers Association has launched a boycott:* Karnowski, "Organic Dairy Growth," and Organic Consumers Association (see www.organicconsumers.org, viewed August 2006).

120 Welfare of beef cattle: Farm Sanctuary, *The Welfare of Cattle in Beef Production: A Summary of the Scientific Evidence.*

121 *the average cow will consume:* See Schlosser, 150.

121 *In the 1950s, farmers began using growth hormones:* Michael Roberts, "U.S. Animal Agriculture: Making the Case for Productivity," *AgBioForum* 3, 2–3 (2002): 120–26. (see www.agbioforum.org/v3n23/v3n23a08-roberts .htm, viewed August 2006).

121 *Cattle on the range:* Jessica Fender, "Ranchers Try to Save Livestock from Flood," *Baton Rouge Advocate,* September 27, 2005, and USDA, 2004 U.S. Animal Health Report, Agriculture Information Bulletin No. 798, APHIS, August 2005.

121 *Cattle may be transported several times:* Farm Sanctuary, *The Welfare of Cattle in Beef Production.*

122 *Every year, many thousands of cattle and calves die in transit:* Temple Grandin, "Livestock Management Practices That Reduce Injuries to Livestock During Transport," *Livestock Trucking Guide,* revised September 2001 (see www .animal-agriculture.org/pamphlets/Livestock%20Trucking/LTG.asp, viewed August 2006).

122 *There's a final indignity:* See Schlosser, 173, and Joby Warwick, "They Die Piece by Piece," *Washington Post,* April 10, 2001.

125 *That particular jump got her out of the slaughter line:* Susan Vela, "Animal Escapades Offered Year Full of Lessons, Reflections for All," *Cincinnati Enquirer,* December 31, 2002.

CHAPTER NINE: IT'S NOT WILBUR'S FARM ANYMORE

129 Welfare of pigs on factory farms: Farm Sanctuary, *The Welfare of Sows in Gestation Crates: A Summary of the Scientific Evidence.*

129 *The animals have disappeared from sight:* Matthew Scully, "A Sunless Hell: Confronting the Cruel Facts of Factory-Farmed Meat," *Arizona Republic,* February 19, 2006.

130 *They won a judgment of $5 million:* Claudia Dreifus, "A Conversation with Robert D. Hall: The Fine Art of Watching a Bug's Life to Explain a Death," *New York Times,* January 2, 2007.

130 *For years, animal welfare scientists have discussed this "repetitive, useless behav-*

ior": Bernard E. Rollin, *Farm Animal Welfare Social, Bioethical, and Research Issues* (Ames: Iowa State University Press, 1995). 40

131   *Near the end of her four-month pregnancy, a sow is moved:* Robert E. Taylor and Thomas G. Field, *Scientific Farm Animal Production.* (Upper Saddle River, N.J.: Prentice-Hall, 1998).

132   *Mortality rates for piglets in these systems are high:* Lewis W. Smith, "Observing Swine Behavior to Lower Piglet Mortality," *Agricultural Research*, June 2001.

132   *On commercial farms, a piglet's life cycle follows a prescribed pattern:* Merle Cunningham and Duane Acker, *Animal Science and Industry,* 6th ed. (Upper Saddle River, N.J.: Prentice Hall 2001), and Plate D, "Swine Production" (after chapter 6 ends on page 140).

132   Boar "milking" and actions "a lot more intimate": Grandin and Johnson, 103.

133   Smithfield Circle employees quit and related conditions they had seen, and Sundberg quote: Brent Israelsen, "Circle Four (Hog Farm) Workers Quit, Decry 'Inhumane' Conditions in Utah Hog Production Factory," *Salt Lake Tribune*, January 30, 2003.

134   Bob Herbert on Smithfield's Tar Heel, North Carolina, pork processing plant: Bob Herbert, "Where the Hogs Come First," *New York Times,* June 15, 2006.

135   American Veterinary Medical Association study of two housing systems for sows: American Veterinary Medical Association (AVMA), Task Force on the Housing of Pregnant Sows, June 2005 (see www.avma.org/about_avma/governance/hod/2005proceedings/2.f.pdf, viewed September 2006).

136   Food Marketing Institute and the National Council of Chain Restaurants voluntary guidelines on welfare of pigs and later statement: Food Marketing Institute (FMI), National Council of Chain Restaurants (NCCR), Report: FMI-NCCR Animal Welfare Program, January 2003.

139   Information on Milgram's experiments: See www.stanleymilgram.com, viewed July 2006.

140   Henry David Thoreau quote: Ellen Hansen, ed., *The New England Transcendentalists: Life of the Mind and of the Spirit* (Lowell, Mass.: Discovery Enterprises, 1993), 26.

142   *Unfortunately, the AVMA has barely changed its attitudes since then:* For information on the American Veterinary Medical Association annual meeting, see www.farmedanimalwatch.org (viewed July 2006).

143   Charlotte's Web plot summary: E. B. White, *Charlotte's Web* (New York: Harper, 1952).

143 *White spared his pig the chopping block:* See excerpts from White's essay, "Saving a Pig's Life," on www.factmonster.com (viewed July 2006).

145 *Between 1999 and 2005, goat meat consumption in the United States rose:* "America's Booming Goat Industry: No Kidding," *The Economist,* August 27, 2005.

145 Numbers of goats being raised in the United States for meat, milk, and mohair: National Agricultural Statistics Service (NASS), Sheep and Goats, USDA, Washington, D.C. Released January 28, 2005 (see http://usda.mannlib.cornell.edu/reports/nassr/livestock/pgg-bb/shep0105.txt, viewed August 2006).

146 *Texas is the leading goat-producing state, followed by Tennessee and California:* National Agricultural Statistics Service (NASS). Sheep and Goats, 2005.

146 *domestic supply cannot meet the demand, so the United States imports more than seventeen million pounds of goat meat each year from Australia and New Zealand:* Marvin Shurley and Frank Craddock, "U.S. Meat Goat Industry: Past, Present and Future," presented at the Gathering of Goat Producers IV, Seguin, Texas, 2005 (see www.theikga.org/us_meat_goat_industry.htm, viewed September 2006).

146 *In 2004, the head of a dairy goat association was charged with mistreating animals:* "Man Charged with Torturing His Goats," Associated Press, posted on WKMG (Central Florida) Local6.com, January 17, 2004.

CHAPTER TEN: THE PECKING DISORDER

147 *Over the past two decades, the number of chickens raised for human consumption:* American Meat Institute (AMI), AMI Fact Sheet: Overview of U.S. Meat and Poultry Production and Consumption, March 2005. For more on the welfare of battery hens, see Farm Sanctuary, *The Welfare of Hens in Battery Cages: A Summary of the Scientific Evidence.*

149 *fertilized eggs are placed in drawers stacked in ceiling-high incubators:* Tyson, "Live Production: Chicken" (see www.tyson.com/Corporate/AboutTyson/LiveProduction/Chicken.aspx, viewed August 2006).

149 *Approximately 300 million layer hens are used in commercial egg production in the United States:* USDA, *Agricultural Statistics 2006* (Washington, D.C.: U.S. Government Printing Office, 2006), VIII-38.

151 Use of arsenic in chicken feed: David Wallinga, "Frequently Asked Questions on Playing Chicken: Avoiding Arsenic in Your Meat," Institute for Agriculture and Trade Policy (see www.iatp.org and www.environmentalobservatory.org, viewed September 2006), and PR Newswire, "Lundy & Davis: Something Fowl in the Air; Research Finds Toxic Contamination From Poultry Industry Linked to Disease and Death," January 10, 2003.

151 *The ammonia in bird feces affects the birds as well:* M. Akan et al., "A Case of Aspergillosis in a Broiler Breeder Flock," *Avian Disease* 46, 2 (2002): 497–501 (see www.ncbi.nlm.nih.gov/entrez/query.fcgi?db=pub med&cmd=Retrieve&dopt=AbstractPlus&list_uids=12061665&query_ hl=2&itool=pubmed_docsum, viewed August 2006). Also R. Korbel, J. Bauer, and B. Gedek, "Pathologico-anatomic and Mycotoxicologic Studies of Aspergillosis in Birds," *Tierarztliche Praxis* 21, 2 (1993): 134–39 (see www.ncbi.nlm.nih.gov/entrez/query.fcgi?itool=abstractplus&db=pubmed &cmd=Retrieve&dopt=abstractplus&list_uids=7832725, viewed August 2006).

152 *for each thousand birds, workers are paid about two dollars:* See Nierenberg, 19.

153 *Studies have shown that large numbers of birds are injured:* See Inma Estevez, "Poultry Welfare Issues," *Poultry Digest Online* 3, 2 (2002) (see www.wattnet .com/library/DownLoad/PD2aw.pdf, viewed September 2006).

155 *layer hens' bodies have been profoundly manipulated and pushed to produce an extraordinary 265 eggs a year, many times the number they would naturally lay:* "General Poultry Information: Nomenclature, Eggs and Tidbits of Information," Avian Sciences, Purdue University (see http://ag.ansc.purdue.edu/ poultry/chickzone/geninfo.htm, viewed August 2006). Also Compassion in World Farming (CIWF), "Facts About Irish Farm Animals—Egg Laying Hens & Egg Labelling" (see www.ciwf.ie/farminfo/farmfacts_egghens.html, viewed August 2006). Also Glasgow Zoo Park, "Poultry" (www.glasgowzoo .co.uk/articles/birds/poultry.php, viewed August 2006).

157 *One slaughter plant can unload and kill more than five thousand birds an hour per slaughter line:* J. M. Sparrey and P. J. Kettlewell, "Shackling of Poultry: Is It a Welfare Problem?" *World's Poultry Science Journal,* July 1994, 167–76.

158 Workers' health risks: See, for example, Melissa Hendricks, "Ellen Silbergeld: Resistance Fighter," *Johns Hopkins Public Health,* spring 2002 (see www.jhsph .edu/Publications/Spring02/features.htm, viewed August 2006).

158   *incredibly, some are still alive and conscious. USDA records show that millions of chickens are boiled alive every year:* USDA, FSIS, Electronic Reading Room: "Animal Disposition Reporting System (ADRS), Chickens Condemned Postmortem in USDA Inspected Establishments, Period: Fiscal Year 2002" (see www.fsis.usda.gov/ophs/adrsdata/2002/pmckfy02.htm, viewed September 2005).

158   *Disease and contamination also go unnoticed:* Data on incidence of salmonella contamination, where it has been found, deaths, and costs, from the USDA's Food Safety Research Information Office, the USDA's Food Safety and Inspection Service, and the USDA's Economic Research Service, cited in "Foul Fowl: An Analysis of Salmonella Contamination in Broiler Chickens," *Food and Water Watch*, July 2006 (see www.foodandwaterwatch.org, viewed July 2006).

159   Virgil Butler experiences and quotes: "Whistleblower on the Kill Floor: An Interview with Virgil Butler and Laura Alexander," *Satya*, February 2006.

160   Benjamin Franklin letter to his daughter, January 26, 1784: Excerpt posted on www.greatseal.com, viewed July 2006.

163   *In 2005, about 256 million turkeys were raised in the United States:* U.S. Census Bureau, "Facts for Features—Thanksgiving Day, November 24, 2005" (see www.census.gov, viewed July 2006).

164   James Cromwell quote: Cliff Rothman, "For His Turkey Day Meal, 'Babe' Actor Cromwell Gobbles Only Vegetables," *USA Today*, November 17, 1998.

164   *the federation arranged to send the turkeys to Disneyland:* Matthew Jones, "Pardoned Turkeys' Next Stop: They're Going to Disneyland," *Virginian Pilot*, November 23, 2005.

CHAPTER ELEVEN: UNNATURAL DISASTERS

167   Death toll of Hurricane Katrina: "Death Toll from Katrina Likely Higher Than 1,300," Associated Press, February 10, 2006, and Anne Kornblutt and Adam Nossiter, "Bush, Returning to New Orleans, Repeats Aid Vow," *New York Times*, August 30, 2006. People forced to evacuate: See Axel Graumann et al., *Hurricane Katrina: A Climatological Perspective*, National Oceanic and Atmospheric Administration, U.S. Department of Commerce, October 2005, updated January 2006.

167   *the economic consequences of Katrina totaled nearly $100 billion:* Graumann et al., *Hurricane Katrina.*

168   *Untold millions of other farmed animals—the vast majority of them chickens—in Alabama, Florida, Georgia, Louisiana, and Mississippi:* An estimate of hundreds of millions of farmed animals in the hurricane zone was produced by the Humane Society of the United States from annual industry production figures (see www.hsus.org/farm_animals/farm_animals_news/farm_animals_ after_katrina.html, viewed September 2006).

168   But more than six million farmed animals, mostly chickens, had lost their lives: "Impact of Hurricane Katrina on Mississippi Agriculture by Mississippi State University Extension Service" (http://msucares.com/pubs/misc/m1426 .pdf, viewed 10/9/07).

168   *In the 1930s, Tyson began operations in the American South:* Human Rights Watch, *Blood, Sweat, and Fear: Workers' Rights in U.S. Meat and Poultry Plants,* 2005, www.hrw.org.

168   *Mississippi alone accounts for 10 percent of U.S. broiler production:* "Poultry Industry Hit Hard by Katrina," *Poultry Health Report,* summer 2005, National Institute for Animal Agriculture (see www.animalagriculture.org, viewed July 2006).

168   Sanderson Farms' market share and sales: See www.sandersonfarms.com, viewed July 2006.

168   Destruction data for broiler chickens in Mississippi killed when sheds destroyed: *Poultry Health Report,* summer 2005.

169   Cows faced starvation: Farm Sanctuary, "Hurricane Katrina Farm Animal News and Rescue Efforts: The Road to Recovery" (see www.farmsanctuary .org/adopt/rescue_hurricane.htm, viewed August 2006).

173   Rooster "rapist-murderers": Grandin and Johnson, 69.

174   Tornadoes and impact on Buckeye Egg Farm: Ohio History Central, Online Encyclopedia, "Buckeye Egg Farm" (see www.ohiohistorycentral.org/entry .php?rec=1672, viewed August 2006.) Also "An Unnatural Disaster," *Farm Sanctuary News,* winter 2001 (www.farmsanctuary.org/newsletter/disaster .htm).

175   Hurricane Floyd in 1999 and hog factory manure lagoons' pollution: Peter T. Kilborn, "Hurricane Reveals Flaws in Farm Law," *New York Times,* October 17, 1999.

175   *Lagoons of hog manure had burst on that occasion, contaminating drinking water and killing vast numbers of fish:* EPA-821-B-01-001, Environmental Assess-

ment of Proposed Revisions to the National Pollutant Discharge Elimination System Regulation and the Effluent Guidelines for Concentrated Animal Feeding Operations, January 2001.

176 Concern about antibiotic resistance and Tollefson quote: Tamar Nordenberg, U.S. Food and Drug Administration, "Miracle Drugs vs. Super Bugs: Preserving the Usefulness of Antibiotics," *FDA Consumer Magazine*, November–December 1998 (see www.fda.gov/fdac/features/1998/698_bugs.html, viewed August 2006).

176 Antibiotic use quoted from Levy: Stuart B. Levy, "What Can We Do to Reduce Antibiotic Resistance?" PBS Roundtable: The Evolving Enemy, 2001 (see www.pbs.org/wgbh/evolution/survival/enemy/index.html, viewed September 2006).

176 Evolution of virulent bacterial resistance and Smith quote: "Superbug Beats Superdrug," BBC News, February 17, 1999 (see http://news.bbc.co.uk/l/hi/health/background_briefings/antibiotics/281632.stm, viewed August 2006).

176 Bird flu mutated most virulently between 1918 and 1919; millions died worldwide: See Greger, *Bird Flu*.

177 Agribusiness and bird flu sources, and animal health experts dispute hypothesis: Leon Bennun, "Reality Takes Wing over Bird Flu," *Viewpoint*, BBC News, February 17, 2006 (see www.bbc.co.uk, viewed August 2006).

177 Virulent strains of bird flu most likely evolved in domesticated poultry, and Ip position: Deborah Silver, "Bird Flu May Be Spreading via Plane, Fish Farm," *Poultry News*, Meatingplace.com, December 29, 2005.

177 Greger research: See Greger, *Bird Flu*.

177 Evolving industry perspectives on bird flu and possible role of infected poultry litter: Silver, "Bird Flu."

178 *A number of people are now confirmed to have died from avian flu . . . ; evidence that human-to-human transmission:* Elisabeth Rosenthal and Donald G. McNeil Jr., "Human-to-Human Infection by Bird Flu Virus Is Confirmed," *New York Times,* June 24, 2006. See also Greger, *Bird Flu*.

178 The National Chicken Council declared September 2005 "National Chicken Month," and situation for broilers and fryers a week after Katrina: USDA, *Broiler Market News Report,* September 6, 2005.

179 Livestock and global warming: H. Steinfeld, et al., *Livestock's Long Shadow: Environmental Issues and Options* (Rome: Food and Agriculture Organization of the United Nations, 2006).

179   Henning Steinfeld quote: "Livestock a Major Threat to Environment," Food and
      Agriculture Organization of the United Nations, press release, November 29, 2006.

CHAPTER TWELVE: IN THE EYES OF THE LAW

187   *This has happened even though, "[f]rom a statistician's point of view . . . all animals
      are farmed animals":* David J. Wolfson and Mariann Sullivan, "Foxes in the Hen
      House: Animals, Agribusiness, and the Law: A Modern American Fable," in
      Cass R. Sunstein and Martha Nussbaum, eds., *Animal Rights: Current Debates
      and New Directions* (New York: Oxford University Press, 2004), 206.

191   Court decision granting Farm Sanctuary standing: In the Court of Appeal of
      the State of California, Second Appellate District, Division One, *Farm Sanc-
      tuary v. Department of Food and Agriculture,* April 22, 1998, 7.

191   Eisenberg quote on appellate court decision: Personal correspondence be-
      tween Sheldon Eisenberg and Gene Baur, March 23, 2007.

194   A single bird needs 303 square inches: "Developing Science-Based Animal Welfare
      Guidelines" by J. A. Mench of U. C. Davis and J. C. Swanson of Kansas State
      University.

195   Egert quote on legal judgment in Wegmans case: Personal correspondence
      between Len Egert and Gene Baur, August 14, 2006.

197   Senator Byrd quote from speech on the U.S. Senate floor: Senator Robert Byrd,
      "Cruelty to Animals," U.S. Senate, July 9, 2001 (see www.nal.usda.gov/awic/
      farmanimals/byrd.htm, viewed August 2006).

200   Wolfgang Puck quote: Kim Severson, "Celebrity Chef Announces Strict
      Animal-Welfare Policy," *New York Times,* March 22, 2007.

206   *"It's gustatory narcissism. . . . What are we willing to do for this flavor?":* Martha
      T. Moore, "Foes See Foie Gras as a Fat Target," *USA Today,* June 5, 2006.

CHAPTER THIRTEEN: BENEATH THE SKIN

209   Details from "Bodies . . . the Exhibition": See www.bodiestheexhibition.com,
      viewed July 2006.

210   American Public Health Association call for a moratorium on new factory farms:
      American Public Health Association, *Association News,* 2003 Policy Statements.

211 *spread of CAFOs was putting the culture of family farming and the environment at risk;* Ohio Farmers' Union representative quote: Tom Henry, "Union Officers Tell Audience Big Operations Hurt Farming," *Toledo Blade,* August 1, 2006.

211 *In 2005, the state of Oklahoma sued poultry operations for pollution from their facilities that had fouled the Illinois River water basin:* Andrew Martin, "Fowl Runoff Spurs Fierce Poultry Fight," *Chicago Tribune,* June 13, 2006.

212 *organic cropland doubled between 1992 and 1997 and, for many crops, doubled again between 1997 and 2003:* USDA, Economic Research Service, Data Sets: Organic Production, updated November 16, 2005 (see www.ers.usda.gov, viewed August 2006).

212 *Sales of organic poultry and dairy have increased by about 20 percent each year since 1997:* USDA, Economic Research Service, 2005.

212 *during the same period, sales of all food in the United States rose only 2 to 4 percent a year:* Organic Trade Association, "Food Facts," Organic Trade Association's 2004 Manufacturer Survey (see www.ota.com, viewed August 2006).

212 *In 2005, sales of organic foods in the United States were nearly $14 billion. That's about 2.5 percent of the total retail market for food:* Organic Trade Association, Organic Trade Association's 2006 Manufacturer Survey, cited in The O'Mama Report, www.theorganicreport.com, viewed August 2006.

212 *just a fraction of the astounding $894 billion Americans spent on food in 2005:* USDA, Economic Research Service, Food CPI, Prices and Expenditures: Food Expenditures by Families and Individuals as a Share of Disposable Personal Income, updated June 9, 2006 (see www.ers.usda.gov, viewed August 2006).

213 A recent article on product labeling spin: Kim Severson, "Be It Ever So Homespun, There's Nothing Like Spin," *New York Times,* January 3, 2007.

213 Cornucopia Institute lawsuit: Cornucopia Institute, "Cornucopia Institute Requests Full USDA Investigation of Alleged Organic Violations at Texas Factory Dairy Farm," press release, July 21, 2006 (see www.cornucopia.org, viewed August 2006).

213 John Mackey quote: Marian Burros, "Does Organic Imply Grazing?" *New York Times,* September 14, 2005.

219 *"Well-planned vegan and other types of vegetarian diets are appropriate for all stages of the life cycle":* American Dietetic Association, Dietitians of Canada, "Position of the American Dietetic Association and Dietitians of Canada: Vegetarian Diets," *Journal of the American Dietetic Association* 103, 6 (2003): 748–65.

221 *over the last thirty years our spending on fast food has increased a staggering eighteen times, from $6 billion to $110 billion a year:* Figure of $6 billion from *Res-
taurants USA,* February 1999. Figure of $110 billion and increased spending
from National Restaurant Association, 2001 Restaurant Industry Forecast,
both cited in Alliance for a Healthier Generation, "Facts and Figures," www
.healthiergeneration.org, viewed July 2006.

221 *in 1930, nearly one-third of Americans' income was used to purchase food:* USDA,
Economic Research Service, updated June 9, 2006.

223 *Estimates suggest that the direct costs of treating obesity-related conditions in the
United States are $117 billion every year and headed higher:* American Heart
Association, "Heart Disease and Stroke Statistics—2006 Update," cited in
Alliance for a Healthier Generation, "Facts and Figures."

Acknowledgments

I am indebted to many people without whom this book would not exist. First of all, a heartfelt thank-you to Mia MacDonald of Brighter Green and Martin Rowe of Lantern Books for working closely with me to craft this manuscript. I appreciate their dedication, clear thinking, creativity, attention to detail, and interest in and concern for the issues explored in the book.

I am grateful as well to my agent, Tracy Brown, my editor, Michelle Howry, and to the whole team at Simon and Schuster, including Trish Todd, Lisa Considine, and my acquiring editor, Nancy Hancock, for the incredible skill and dedication they brought to the project. Tracy and Michelle in particular have shepherded the book along, and Tracy has provided key support throughout the entire process.

My friend Matthew Scully contributed wise counsel and helpful edits, and I thank both Matthew and Emmanuelle Scully for their help and hospitality during the writing of the book. Lauren Ornelas also provided essential support, perspective, advice, and edits throughout. I'm deeply grateful to Lauren for that and so much more. Others who helped with research, input, and other assistance include: Renada Beranek, Chloe Jo Berman, Michelle DeBlaere, Rebekah Mullaney, Nicolette Hahn Niman, Miyun Park, Matt Prescott, Samantha Ragsdale, Tricia Barry, Norm Scott, Paul Shapiro, and Kate Travaline. And I'm grateful to Susie Coston, Farm Sanctuary's shelter director, who supplied many of the animal stories; Jeff Lydon, our executive director, who reviewed the manuscript; and Mariann Sullivan, an attorney and Farm Sanctuary board member who gave important advice on the chapter about laws.

Working in animal protection over the years, I've come to know a pretty remarkable group of people, including Carol Adams, Holly Cheever, Joyce D'Silva, Bruce Friedrich, Lorin Lindner, Jim Mason, Tom and Nancy Regan, Peter Singer, Kim Sturla, Will Tuttle, Zoe Weil, the late Henry Spira, artist Sue Coe, attorney David Wolfson, and my longtime friend Wayne Pacelle, now president and CEO of the Humane Society of the United States. When confronting animal cruelty, you don't always see the best in humanity, but friends like these have always been a reminder to me of the dedication, idealism, and compassion of which human beings are capable.

I am profoundly grateful as well to the many good-hearted people and organizations who have helped Farm Sanctuary since its founding in the 1980s. The list runs long, and even then it's only partial. It includes: Jennifer Abbot, Ahimsa Foundation, Grant Aleksander, Nanci Alexander, Diane and Tom Anderson, Animal Welfare Trust, John Archibald, Archibald Family Foundation, Joy Askew, Teri Barnato, Dennis and Stacey Barsema, Lorri Bauston, Dorr Begnal, Valerie Belt, Bill Bey, Laurelee Blanchard, Melissa Bonfiglio, Bosack and Kruger Charitable Foundation, Jody Boyman, Berkeley Breathed, John Broderick, Audrey Burnand, Linda Buyukmihci-Bey, Pam and Jerry Cesak, Michele and Agnese Cestone Foundation, Trish Chilbert, Jamie Cohen, Joseph Connelly, James Costa, Marilyn Crawford, Leanne Cronquist, Cory Wade Curdt, Jeanne and Ed Daniels, Stewart and Terri David, Davy Davidson, Karen Dawn, Orly Degani, Antonia Demas, Todd and Denise Denlinger, Len Egert, George Eisman, Dennis Erdman, Fred Ey, Mary Finelli, Mitchell Fox, Frankenberg Foundation, Lester Friedlander, Kathryn Fugere, Sharon Gannon, Priscilla and Mickey Gargalis, Kirstie Gholson, Caryn Ginsberg, Dan Ginsburg, Glaser Progress Foundation, Colleen Patrick Godreau, Brad and Sunny Goldberg, Derek Goodwin, Nancy Gordon, Che Green, Michael Greger, Andrea Gullo, Paul Harvey Jr., Lara and Mark Heiman, Jane Hoffman, Robin Ishmael, Julie Janovsky, Anne-Claire and Lionel Jolivot, Dena Jones, Harold and Garland Jones, Satish Karandikar, Blanche Kent, Chris Kerr, Michael Klaper, Jana Kohl, Larry Kopp, Allene LaPides, Ador Lazar, Emily Levine, Emily Libla, David Life, Barb and Greg Lomow, Lawrence Carter Long, Sally Mackler, Grace and Mike Markarian, Jeffrey Moussaieff Masson, Mary and Peter Max, Jo McArthur, Susan McBride, Patrick McDonnell, Holly McNulty, Sean McVity, Kathy Meyer, Gil Michaels, Ken Midkiff, Cheryl Miller, Diane Miller, Marisa Miller, Jane Valez Mitchell, Keith Mohler, Sandra Mohr, Nicole Montalbano, Carol Moon, Laura Moretti, Jane Morrison, Steve Murray, Gina Myers, Mike Myers, Nalith, Inc., Susan Nauslar, Lewis

Neiman, Jeff and Sabrina Nelson, Kari Nienstedt, Karen O'Connell, Susan and Bill O'Connell, Teresa Ohmit, Park Foundation, Folke H. Peterson Foundation, Tanya Petrovna, John Phillips, Dan Piraro, The Prentice Foundation, Inc., Sherry Ramsey, Meg and Lewis Randa, Dawn Ratcliff, Stephanie and Paul Rebein, Katherine Reiser, Warren Reynolds, Jonathan Richmond, Terrin and Erik Riemer, Heathcliff Rothman, Shelly Schleuter, Tom Scholz, Don and Elaine Sloan, Ashley Lou Smith, Mariana and Robert Steele, Peter Stevenson, Allison Stoll, Paul Swedenburg, John Talbot, Deborah Tanzer, Margaretta Taylor, Joyce Tischler, Marlene and Larry Titus, Michael Tobias, Tortuga Foundation, Joey Trackman, Amy Trakinski, Cathy Unruh, Bernie Unti, Heather and Leor Veleanu, Sonia and Pablo Waisman, Paul Waldau, Bob and June Warren, Kathy White, Persia White, Roger White, Tracy and Noah Wyle, the late Gretchen Wyler, and the Youth Development Foundation.

Finally, a special thanks to my brothers and sisters: Michael, Kathy, Steve, Bonnie, and Lisa. Life has always been better for their company and friendship, and each in their own way has taught me important things. And I will always be grateful to my boyhood companion, Tiger, a cat who touched my heart and taught me how the friendship of animals can enrich our lives.

INDEX

About the Author

GENE BAUR grew up in Hollywood, California, where he worked as an extra in television, films, and commercials, including several spots for McDonalds and other fast-food chains. It was during college at California State University, Northridge, when he first started becoming active in animal issues. In 1986 Baur co-founded Farm Sanctuary, which has grown into America's leading farm animal protection organization. Baur and his Farm Sanctuary colleagues have rescued hundreds of live animals left for dead at stockyards and slaughterhouses—and his pictures and videos exposing the cruelties of factory farming have been aired nationally and internationally. Baur has testified before Congress and many state legislatures, and his organization has initiated groundbreaking legal reforms to prevent farm animal abuse. The efforts of Farm Sanctuary have been covered by leading news organizations, including the *New York Times, Los Angeles Times, Wall Street Journal, Washington Post,* National Public Radio, ABC, NBC, CBS, and CNN. Baur is a resident of Watkins Glen, New York.

Farm Sanctuary

Discussion Points

1. What were the larger societal trends that fostered a transition from traditional, independent farm work to factory farming? Do you believe these transitions toward factory farming are inevitable signs of progress? Why or why not?

2. Which of the animal profiles proved most memorable for you? Why? Why do you believe Baur employs the animal profile? What are his aims? Do you believe he is successful? Why or why not?

3. How does the author's reference to animals as individuals, sentient beings, units of production, and meat impact your understanding of the power and value of labels? What do you perceive to be the primary challenge in engaging the public in reimagining the labels we attach to animals raised for food?

4. What are downers? How do Baur and his fellow advocates use their plight to spur changes at the Lancaster Stockyards? What were the gains and losses in their first major animal rights campaign?

5. What are the compelling images for you as Baur recounts the life of the animals on either Watkins Glen or the Orland, California, sanctuary? In evaluating these images, what strikes you as a departure or a new facet in your own thinking? To what do you attribute this change? What impact do you imagine it will have on your behavior, if any?

6. Describe what Baur calls the "bigger is better" mentality that exists in agribusiness. Do you see evidence of this mentality in other business arenas? If so, where? If not, why does it exist in agribusiness

alone? What do you believe underlies the pursuit for bigger? Can this mentality be challenged successfully? If yes, provide examples of arenas where this has occurred. If not, why not?

7. What does Baur mean by the term *pigmanship*? How does his understanding of the value of this term evolve throughout the course of the book? What do you believe are potential synonyms for this term?

8. As we uncover the practices of meat production for a variety of animals, a clear pattern emerges across cow, sheep, chicken, and even egg production. Illuminate this pattern and the arguments Baur uses to challenge agribusiness owners' contention that animal behavior necessitate their practices. Do you foresee a potential middle ground between these two perspectives? Why or why not?

9. Identify the natural behaviors of the following animals: pigs, cows, chickens, and sheep. Do many of their behaviors coincide with your own conceptions of these animals? Why or why not?

10. How has Baur's own conception of sanctuary changed from its earlier incarnation at the start of his animal rights work? Why was the change necessary?

A Conversation with Gene Baur

As a teen, you characterized yourself as on a search for a way to integrate your life with your values. To what do you attribute your valuing of animals beyond what some may consider the norm? Were there moments when your ready recognition of animals as individuals waned or was challenged? What were the circumstances? If not, why do you believe you have maintained your valuing of animals so deeply?

I have always been very sensitive and pained to see others, including animals, suffer. But growing up, I didn't think about the animals I was eating, until one day I came home and saw a dead chicken's body, with wings and legs, laying on his or her back, cooked for dinner. I didn't eat meat that night or for a while afterward.

Then, beginning in 1986, I began investigating hundreds of farms, stockyards, and slaughterhouses across the United States to document conditions. Since then, the reality of factory-farming abuse has been seared into my soul. Those painful images, and the wondrous transformations that occur when victims are rescued from that system, have informed and strengthened my deepest convictions. Spending time with farm animals has helped me understand and respect them as individuals.

In your story about Maya, you said very little was known about animal emotions in the 1980s. How has your understanding of animal emotions changed since then? What are some of the major insights in the field? Who are some of the major researchers of animal emotions?

I believe people who live with and pay attention to farm animals, including those of us at Farm Sanctuary, have long recognized these creatures' sentience and emotions. But there has been little institutional attention paid to the topic. Most academic research has dealt with how to more profitably exploit pigs, chickens, cows, and other "food" animals, rather than on how to understand them as individuals. But that is changing. We're coming to understand more about farm animals' emotions and social relationships; their capacities for fear and joy, learning and communicating. Some leaders in the field of animal sentience include Jane Goodall, Marc Bekoff, and Jonathan Balcombe.

As you recount the development of corporate factory farming, you highlight some of the ways that individual farmers are forced to adopt "technological advancements" that challenge individual farmers' own best interests. How do you and others fight the presumption that mechanization or technological innovation is an inevitable rite of passage for progress?

I think we need to carefully assess what is meant by *progress*. Too often, agribusiness measures progress in terms of shortsighted financial gains, commonly at the expense of broader concerns (animal welfare, environmental and economic sustainability, and human health). We need to look at the whole system, with all the related costs and benefits. I think innovation and change, which could include new technology, are natural and inevitable, and they can be positive as long as all the impacts are understood and accounted for. I believe innovation and creativity can help us produce healthy food in an efficient, ecologically sustainable, and compassionate way.

You wrote about the unsuccessful campaign to pass the Downed Animal Protection Act and suggest that the creation of Humane USA will help redress some of the challenges you and others encountered. Can you expound specifically on the lessons you learned from that campaign? How do you think Humane USA can remedy some of the problems the campaign encountered?

Humane USA is a political action committee that is involved in the election process. It plays an important role in supporting animal-friendly legislators and it makes accountable those who hinder the enactment of laws and policies to prevent cruelty. Lawmakers will now face consequences for their actions.

When you look at the success of passing 599f in California, the foie gras battles in California and Chicago and other cities, and Proposition 10 in Florida and Proposition 204 in Arizona, what convergence of factors made these successes possible? What challenges/barriers still exist in ensuring these and other legislative measures continue to be effective?

In all these cases, a clear abuse was identified and made known to a large number of citizens, a simple remedy was proposed, and mechanisms existed for legislation to move forward. In the case of 599f in California and the foie gras laws in California and Chicago, we had strong leadership who worked hard to advance their proposals through the legislative process. In Florida and Arizona, we were able to place issues on the ballot through citizens' initiatives, and in each case, a solid majority voted to ban cruel farming practices.

We'll continue working to advance similar measures in the future, and I believe we'll continue to have success. Among the greatest challenges we face is the wealth and entrenched influence of factory farms who profit from current system, and unwitting consumer participation, apathy, and a tendency to go along with old habits without questioning the status quo.

When I was growing up *veal* was a dirty word even as we continued to eat lots of other meats. Do you foresee some meats more than others

acquiring a tainted image similar to that of veal? Which ones and why? Do you believe it's possible for the meat industry to rehabilitate the image of veal? Why or why not?

I think *veal* became a dirty word because people were made aware of how calves are treated to produce it. Other meats are the result of similar cruelties, and also deserve a tainted image. I believe most people would be appalled to learn how chickens, turkeys, pigs, dairy cows, and other animals are treated to produce meat, milk, and eggs. There will likely be efforts to market veal and other meats as "humane," but these claims should be questioned. Do the words *humane* and *slaughter* fit together?

Based upon your experiences as a student at Cornell, you noted how other students became increasingly desensitized to the plight of animals and took on the values of agribusiness throughout their tenure. How would you rectify this situation if you could have a hand in crafting your own undergraduate or graduate education experience for students?

I think students should be exposed to different points of view, and encouraged to think about whether it's appropriate to subject farm animals to certain conditions. Common assumptions, including the idea that animals are here for our purposes, or that it is healthy and appropriate to slaughter and eat them, should be discussed.

What are the emerging issues in animals' rights in terms of food production for the next ten to twenty-five years? How are you and fellow advocates engaging young people, so they can continue to fight for animal rights in the coming years? What are the issues that seem most compelling for young people?

Increasingly, I think there will be fundamental questions raised about humans' role on earth and if it's appropriate to treat other animals the way we do, including whether we should exploit them for food. As part of Farm Sanctuary's efforts, we are reaching out to students in schools through our humane education program. We also distribute literature, videos, and other educational materials and host various youth events at our farms. Young people seem to have a natural connection with animals and an inherent understanding of their sentience, qualities we hope to nurture and support and propagate.

What is your vision of the best food production practices in the United States? Can you identify foreign models from which we might take inspiration?

I envision a local, diversified, veganic farming system where food is produced by many gardeners and farmers in both urban and rural settings without using any animals or animal products. In cities, food would be grown in community gardens, as well as on rooftops and on windowsills in apartments. In suburban areas with more land, fruit trees and edible landscaping could supply fresh fruits and vegetables. And the rural countryside would be dotted with small farms producing food primarily for local populations.

Historically, people around the world have been closely connected with the land—growing food on community-based, diversified small farms. I'd like to see a return to that kind of farming system, along with techniques like canning and other methods, some traditional and some new and innovative, to add value and provide food beyond the growing season.

If you could encourage readers to take one specific action to aid in animal rights as it pertains to food or meat production, what would that action be? What do you believe would be the potential consequences of this act?

The single most important action each of us can take to aid animals and promote a healthy planet is to become vegan. By choosing not to use animal products (e.g., meat, dairy, eggs, wool, leather, etc.), we do not support and enable industries that exploit other animals. When citizens make conscientious choices and eschew animal products, businesses will make adjustments to meet consumer demand. A shift toward a plant-based food system would bring about vast, positive impacts. Animals wouldn't be exploited, consumers' health would improve, fewer resources (e.g., land, water, fossil fuels) would be expended, both urban and rural communities would be improved, and it would even help arrest global warming.

Enhance Your Book Club Experience

1. Create a Public Service Announcement (PSA) to promote the idea of pigmanship. Sample PSAs can be found here:

   http://www.madd.org/Media-Center/Media-Center/Media-Library/
   PSAs/Television-PSAs.aspx
   http://www.civilrights.org/about/Iccref/programs/psa/
   http://www.aclu.org/multimedia/ads/index.html

   Your PSA can either be in the form of a storyboard, a series of drawings that illuminate exactly what would appear on the television screen for a thirty-second advertisement or a print ad that could be easily found in a magazine or your local newspaper. Consider the most effective PSAs you have encountered in your lifetime or from the above sample web sites and you will see that they grab their viewers'/readers' attention, promote a specific course of action, and provide relevant facts about their particular issue. Similarly, your PSA should do the same for the idea of pigmanship. (Please feel free to share your work with Farm Sanctuary.)

   Prior to meeting to discuss the book, divide your reading group membership into groups of equal members. Each group will present their PSA to the entire membership when you meet to discuss the book. After all groups have presented their PSA, the entire membership should vote by anonymous ballot for the "top" advertisements based upon the following criteria:

   - Which ad presented the clearest idea of pigmanship?
   - Which ad presented an action that can be easily done by the public?
   - Which ad allows the viewer/audience to emotionally connect to pigmanship?
       a) Was there general consensus among the ads? If yes, why? If no, why not?
       b) What were the most surprising, yet revealing interpretations of pigmanship?

2. Create a vegan spread for your reading group meeting using some of the recipes listed below from www.vegforlife.org as recommended by Gene Baur.

Appetizer
TAPENADE (SERVE WITH CRACKERS)

4 oz pitted green olives (1 cup)
4 oz pitted black olives (1 cup)
4 cloves garlic
¼ cup extra virgin olive oil
2 oz sun-dried tomatoes
1 tbs flat leaf parsley
Fine sea salt and freshly ground black pepper, to taste

Combine all ingredients in a food processor or blender. Then season to taste with salt and pepper.

Entrée
MACARONI AND 'CHEESE'

14 oz uncooked elbow macaroni
4 cups water
10 ½ oz package soft silken tofu, drained
1 cup soymilk
½ cup tahini
3 tbs nutritional yeast
1 tsp turmeric
Salt to taste
2 tbs margarinet

Preheat oven to 350 degrees. Boil macaroni in water until just underdone; drain in colander. Run cold water over macaroni to stop cooking. Blend tofu and soymilk in blender or food processor until smooth Add tahini, nutritional yeast, turmeric, and salt; mix until smooth. In a large bowl, stir together macaroni and "cheese" sauce. Place mixture in lightly oiled ovenproof casserole; top with pats of margarine. Bake until golden and bubbly, about 20 minutes. Makes 10 servings.

Per Serving: Calories: 277, protein: 11 g, carbohydrates: 36 g, cholesterol: 0, sodium: 363 mg, fiber: 3 g.

SPAGHETTI WITH MEATY MUSHROOM SAUCE

½ cup textured vegetable protein flakes or granules
½ cup boiling water
8 oz spaghetti
2 tsp olive oil
1 cup chopped onions
2 cloves garlic, minced or pressed
1 cup chopped mushrooms
1 16 oz can tomato sauce (2 cups)
2 tbs tomato paste
2 tbs soy sauce
1 tsp dried basil leaves
½ tsp dried oregano leaves
Salt and ground black pepper, to taste

Place the textured protein in a small, heatproof mixing bowl and pour the boiling water over it. Mix well and set aside.

Fill a 4 ½ -quart saucepan two-thirds full with water. Bring the water to a rolling boil, and cook the pasta in it until it is al dente. Drain the pasta well and return it to the saucepan. Cover the saucepan with a lid and set it aside.

Meanwhile, heat the oil in a 2-quart (or larger) saucepan over medium-high heat. When the oil is hot, add the onion and garlic and sauté them for 10 minutes.

Then add the mushrooms and rehydrated textured protein (from the first step), and sauté them for 5 minutes longer.

Stir in the remaining ingredients, and bring the sauce to a boil. Reduce the heat to medium-low, and simmer the sauce uncovered for 15 minutes, stirring occasionally.

Pour the sauce over the reserved pasta in the saucepan (from the second step). Toss them together well, and serve at once.

Per serving: Calories: 273, protein: 14 g, carbohydrates: 45 g, fat: 4 g
Recipe courtesy Vegan Vittles, Book Publishing Company

Dessert
CHOCOLATE CHIP COOKIES

> *2 ¼ cups flour*
> *1 tsp baking soda*
> *½ tsp salt*
> *½ cup cane sugar or other dry sweetener*
> *¼ cup brown sugar*
> *½ cup margarine*
> *½ cup oil*
> *3 tbs water*
> *1 ½ tsp vanilla extract*
> *1 cup nondairy chocolate chips*
> *½ cup walnuts or pecans*

In a large bowl, mix the flour, baking soda, and salt. Set aside.

In a small bowl, mix together the cane sugar, brown sugar, margarine, oil, water, and vanilla extract until smooth.

Add to the flour mixture in the large bowl and stir to combine.

Add the chocolate chips and nuts and stir.

Preheat oven to 375 degrees.

Drop by the teaspoonful onto an ungreased cookie sheet.

Bake for 8–10 minutes.

3. Using the examples of animal profiles in *Farm Sanctuary* as a guide, create your own version of an animal profile complete with picture to share with other members of your reading group.

Who is the animal in your life?

What are his/her unique qualities?

Describe the circumstances under which s/he came into your life.

What lessons has s/he taught you?

What specific emotions do you believe s/he has demonstrated to you? To others?

What kinds of relationships does s/he have with other animals?

How does s/he communicate her/his needs?

If you do not have an animal in your life, identify a friend or associate who has one in his/her life. Interview this friend/associate and create a profile of his/her significant animal.

Encourage reading group members to display their profiles on a viewing wall prior to the start of the meeting. During a break, peruse other members' animal profiles. Discuss the impact of writing your profile and reading others' profiles.

Did members see their own animals differently as a result of writing the profile? If so, in what ways?

If you profiled a friend's animal, what was that process like? What did you take away from the writing of the profile? What new insights did you gain about your friend? About their animal?

What will members take away from doing this exercise?